ADVANCE PRAISE

This is a fabulous comprehensive strategy to empower individuals who want to take ownership of their healthcare while achieving real savings in the process. The adoption of a few essential practices will help any individual, or family, save money on prescription medication while getting a better understanding of the healthcare system and how it works. The advantage of multiple "real world" examples is priceless.

—KEN ROSE, RPH, RETAIL, MAIL, AND MANAGED CARE
PHARMACY EXPERT, (THIRTY-SEVEN-PLUS YEARS)

Having taught thousands of individuals to recognize and identify those stress-inducing moments, and then break free from the sometimes harmful impact of stress, this book offers individuals a great leg up in managing stress related to health issues. The techniques, tools, and transparency turn you from a passive participant to an active driver of your health. When you're engaged and informed, you reduce your stress, make better decisions, and experience better outcomes.

—DR. FRANK WOOD, PHD, PSYCHOLOGIST, AND
FOUNDER OF THRIVING WITH STRESS

Scott's book has been a game-changer for me in terms of how I approach the world of healthcare and insurance. I feel empowered to make the right decisions now, not as confused or passive about these issues as I have in the past. For example, when I signed up for insurance coverage through a new employer this summer, I understood how to choose a plan right for me instead of just automatically opting for the lowest deductible. I knew what questions to ask and what to look for when reviewing plan information. Plus, I wasn't afraid to call and ask if something wasn't clear. A couple months later, when I had a procedure done that I knew my insurance would not cover, I negotiated with the provider for a discount because I was paying in cash. None of these would have happened had I not read Healthcare Is Making Me Sick, which taught me how to be a consumer of healthcare—and it can do the same for you.

—JESSICA BURDG, REAL-LIFE HEALTHCARE CONSUMER

HEALTHCARE IS MAKING ME SICK

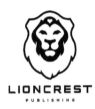

LIONCREST

PUBLISHING

HEALTHCARE IS MAKING ME SICK

Learn the Rules to Regain Control and Fight for Your Healthcare

ISBN   978-1-5445-1197-9 *Paperback*

978-1-5445-1196-2 *Ebook*

To all of those who have been overwhelmed and bewildered by our healthcare and health insurance options. To those of you lost, anxious, and feeling stressed about how you can both provide for your health/well-being and figure out how to pay for it. To all of you who are fed up and are willing to a plot different course. My hope is that this book helps you start that journey.

CONTENTS

DISCLAIMER

The Healthcare market is dynamic and ever-changing. Representations, statistics, websites, and contacts in this book are presented on an "as is" basis at the time of writing, and will change over time.

The views, thoughts, and opinions expressed in this book belong solely to the author.

Any action you take upon the information in this book is strictly at your own choosing and risk.

CHAPTER ONE

DOES HEALTHCARE SEEM CONFUSING? THAT ENDS TODAY.

"I'm mad as hell, and I'm not going to take this anymore."

If you've ever seen the movie *Network*, you'll remember veteran TV news anchor Howard Beale yelling this searing sentiment into the camera, calling on citizens to open their windows and yell along with him. Soon windows were opening in cities across the country in solidarity with Beale's message: the world was going crazy, and nobody was talking about it. The refrain caught fire:

"I'm as mad as hell, and I'm not going to take this anymore."

That's how I feel, today, about the current state of

healthcare. I'm mad as hell! Healthcare consumers are so disenfranchised by the healthcare complex—the consortium of politicians, big hospitals, insurance companies, pharmaceutical companies, and even doctors—that they feel powerless to affect change. And they are not (powerless, that is).

To paraphrase Bob Dylan, these times are a'changing! By the end of this book, you WILL be flinging open your windows and yelling along with me, "I don't have to take this anymore."

Here's what I'm going to teach you:

- The difference between health insurance and your healthcare.
- How to become an informed and confident consumer of health insurance and healthcare so you can stretch your dollar and enhance your outcomes.
- How to avoid the healthcare complex by staying healthy.

Along the way, I am going to give you examples and stories which will help you see what I see: you do not have to be in the dark when it comes to this subject; I will give you tools and resources which enable you to be in charge.

Why are the healthcare and the health insurance systems

in this country failing to respond to the voices and needs of so many consumers? Make no mistake: those frantically fiddling with Obamacare or trying to tailor-make a Trumpcare aren't necessarily focused on your end goals, but their own. It's sad but true.

Some people care, of course—doctors, nurses, researchers, other professionals, and volunteers around the country take your health to heart, and most are immensely dedicated and talented. Insurance companies, major medical centers, and big businesses, however, have business interests that aim to turn a profit. Third parties are all negotiating with each other, and the consumer is excluded. Politicians crave and cater to the power of these industries, saying whatever will get them reelected. They preserve their own self interests. The insurance companies and hospital companies are well organized and influential. We are not.

Is the system evil? Are insurance companies bad? Am I condemning politicians? No—they all have ethics, ideals, and motivations that drive them. It's simply human nature to strive to meet your own objectives—you do it, and insurance companies do it, too. In the US healthcare universe of so-called third-party payers, however, it's easy to forget that what *you* decide matters most.

WHAT DO I MEAN BY THIRD-PARTY PLAYERS?

Third-party players are the US government, health insurance companies, and the healthcare providers (hospitals, physicians, and drug companies). They all negotiate with and lobby each other without your input. **Their needs are being met; are yours? You are on the outside but footing the bill. That's why healthcare is failing in the US.**

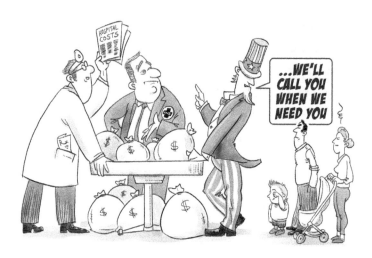

Nobody is responsible for your healthcare but the person you see when you look in the mirror, and you ought to be empowered with the knowledge and tools you need to make the best decisions for yourself and your family. Healthcare isn't a mystery. Nobody is forcing you to write a blank check without understanding your options.

Ready to take back control? Stay with me.

WHY DID I WRITE THIS BOOK, AND WHY SHOULD YOU READ IT?

I decided to write this book for one and only one reason: to help you. I built a business that helped corporations save money on their healthcare costs. I realize healthcare is an enormous problem for many people, and maybe you're one of them. You're confused. You're frustrated. You feel rushed to choose a plan even though you don't truly understand anything beyond the bottom-line deductible and out-of-pocket max. You feel like healthcare and insurance—two vastly different animals—speak a different language, making open dialogue impossible.

Maybe you're angry. Afraid. Despairing or living on the edge of despair. Sick and sad. Feeling like you can't do anything about the cost and the complications of understanding and navigating insurance, providers, and, policy.

I'm here to stop all that. My book flips the script. My agenda is your agenda. You are not helpless when it comes to your healthcare. I am, and will be, your advocate. I intend to cut through the clutter, demystify the myths, correct misinformation, and uncover opportunities you never knew about.

The information in the pages of this book is for first-time

insurance buyers, those in the middle of the journey. In short, it's for any consumer of healthcare—and you *are* a consumer, a topic we'll explore more deeply in chapter 2. Bottom line: it's your health, and if you're not happy with the way things work, it's time you took back your power. I'm going to provide you with a wealth of information—with one caveat. This is not a book full of dry healthcare facts you can't use. Yes, I aim to teach you, but I want those teachings to inspire action, not answer obscure *Jeopardy!* questions. My tone is uncompromising and full of practical steps you can take to put the power back where it belongs: in your hands.

I wrote this book to be a resource, a guide, a map, or a GPS of sorts to help you get back into the driver's seat with your insurance company, employer's benefit program, doctors, labs, drug makers, and pharmacy. When you're done reading, you'll feel empowered and in control of not only your healthcare, but your healthcare dollars. Yes, you read that right: you will be in control of it all, from the type of plan you choose, to how much you pay out-of-pocket, to how you pay for it. You'll find out actual costs of everything from doctor visits to mammograms to major surgeries—and ways to lower those costs by knowing whom to talk to and how to negotiate. You'll discover tools, resources, and techniques that will enhance your healthcare outcomes. And you will hopefully learn that you can make a difference.

How does it all work? You can access methods that will make people hear you because, at the end of the day, they do want your business. You'll be surprised by the incentives and workarounds available if you take the time to look. But remember: you can't be in control of your healthcare if you don't invest the time into understanding it fully, and that's where I come in.

WHY SHOULD YOU LISTEN TO ME?

Who am I, and how am I qualified to offer advice, information, and strategies to streamline and upgrade how you handle your healthcare? Fair question.

Here's the answer: I am an insider. As a consultant who spent twenty-plus years seeking better solutions to problems for clients on the inside of the healthcare, I have worked with pricing, plan design, negotiations, and vendor reviews across a spectrum of clients with varying employee benefit needs. I have an inside perspective. I understand how things work. I know where to find wiggle room. I know tricks of the trade. I can help you with all-important access to information. I will teach you to cut through the noise and insurance jargon and acronyms—what we affectionately call the "alphabet soup of the industry" (HMO, PPO, POS, HRA, HAS, FSA, PCP, and more).

You, on the other hand, are an outsider—but maybe not

for long. My experience getting answers and finding ways to leverage them now applies to *you*. The information I offer is solution-structured, so you can use it wisely. My interest and keen attention is on my readers and improving their lives.

I am taking what I know, offering real-life examples, and providing a menu of recommendations that will make healthcare feel like less of a burden and more of a benefit to you, my readers. After all, you're not a patient; you are a person. You shouldn't be patient, either, because the healthcare industry train is going to keep barreling onward, with or without your input. It's time to slow the train down by providing less fuel (your money) for its engines.

But how?

Many consumer companies are stunned when their product loses market share to a competitor offering what is, to the consumer, an equivalent performance at a much lower price. Think Gillette razors, known by many as a well-regarded but very expensive shave system, and the Dollar Shave Club. Gillette developed the superior Fusion shaving blade, captured most of the market, and charged significantly more for the blades than the previous technology. Enter the Dollar Shave Club. They recognized an opportunity. Although Gillette provided an excellent shave, its new product performance did not necessarily warrant a higher price. Dollar Shave Club produced a similar shaving experience, significantly reduced the price, and enhanced the purchasing experience by mailing it to your house. Men flocked to it. It did not stop with similar technology. Google Trends data blog stated, "Since the razor wars, a conclusion among thinking men has been made; adding more shave tech and blades doesn't equal a better shave, just a lighter wallet. From 2009 to 2014, popularity of classic wet shaving went up 1000 percent! Men have been ditching their plastic, gel-covered, four- and five-bladed heads for the quality, comfort, and savings offered by premium safety and straight razors."[1]

Gillette lost market share and reduced their price to compete effectively. And that's what happens in all markets where the consumer can vote with their own dollar (and walk with their feet)—competition requires companies to adjust to provide a better overall value in the interest of keeping the consumer on their side.

STATS YOU NEED TO KNOW

Gillette saw their market share drop from 70 percent in 2010 to 54 percent in 2016. They retooled their mar-

---

[1] 03, 2018 January. "Did the Razor Wars Spark the Classic Wet Shaving Revolution?" West Coast Shaving. Accessed August 15, 2018. https://www.westcoastshaving.com/blogs/wet-shaving-and-grooming-blog/did-the-razor-wars-spark-the-classic-wet-shaving-revolution.

keting efforts and dropped their prices by 25 percent to compete with newcomers such as Dollar Shave Club.[2]

It should and can work the same way in healthcare. You're the consumer. You shouldn't have to pay high prices for minor outcome enhancement in healthcare. If you make different choices, you'll soon see better products on the shelf and/or encourage competition to reduce pricing on existing services.

The Nexium and Prilosec drug evolution is an example of this dynamic in prescription medicine. Both Prilosec and Nexium treat the same condition (gastrointestinal ailments such as acid reflux), and both are manufactured by AstraZeneca. Nexium, the newer of the two, was purported to be more effective than Prilosec and, when marketed as the "Purple Pill" was priced four to eight times that of Prilosec. But was the "Purple Pill" worth that price upcharge?

Not at all. In fact, meta-studies showed the two drugs used essentially the same active ingredient with very little clinical difference between the two when dosed similarly. And that was the rub—Nexium's superiority over Prilosec

2   Heath, Thomas. "How Hipster Brands Have the King of Razors on the Run." The Washington Post. April 05, 2017. Accessed April 04, 2018. https://www.washingtonpost.com/business/capitalbusiness/how-hipster-brands-have-the-king-of-razors-on-the-run/2017/04/05/edca3af6-1a27-11e7-9887-1a5314b56a08_story.html?utm_term=.c755e774e3c0.

was based on a *40mg* dose of Nexium versus a *20mg* dose of Prilosec.

An informed healthcare consumer could take two generic Prilosec at a *fraction* of the cost of one "Purple Pill" and achieve equivalent relief.[3]

This book will show you how your healthcare and health insurance works—and, above all, how to leverage that knowledge into action. My website, **Uncoveredhc.com,** will continue the journey, providing timely updates to navigate the healthcare and health insurance mazes.

Similarly, I am going to show you how to become a better healthcare and health insurance consumer. My method is easy to follow and has a great likelihood of success—but (and it's a big but) my commitment is not to help you slice your costs in half. That is not viable, and I don't make promises I can't keep. I am certain, however, that I can help you find programs and approaches that fit your goals and thus provide better outcomes at better costs, but not without the essential ingredient: your involvement and devotion to doing something bold. It won't always be easy. If you take this journey, though, you'll see a difference. And you'll see that difference can be made with what is at the end of your arms: your own hands!

---

3   "FREQUENTLY ASKED QUESTIONS - SAMHSA." Accessed September 6, 2018. https://www. samhsa.gov/sites/default/files/faqs-applying-confidentiality-regulations-to-hie.pdf.

A HEFTY DOSE OF TOUGH LOVE

No doubt: I am offering a heavy dose of tough love. The momentous move to take back control of your healthcare is less of a choice and more of an imperative if we are going to bring collective change to an industry in which so many people are simply treading water because they don't know they're allowed to swim. Action is the only choice that can bring change for you and almost everyone you know. We must create a movement; there is power in numbers. We can all become crusaders for change and propel a healthcare consumer revolution, much like the way the Carfax app and similar apps helped revolutionize buying cars by prioritizing transparency. You can use the app for everything from price ranges to whether or not a prospective car has been in an accident. Carfax and others' foray into transparency motivated car manufacturers to embrace transparency. Today you can visit Ford, GM, Toyota, and others to see transparent pricing with all available discounts and inventory across the country. In other words, the power of transparency and information is literally in your hands! Why can't healthcare be the same? It should! But the planting, the weeding, and the harvesting—the homework—is triggered by your effort. Your enthusiastic commitment to that effort is essential.

The transparency in the car market has exploded! Carfax, CarMax, Auto Trader, Edmunds, True Car, Cars.com, Used Car Search Pro, Auto List Car Buying Guide—they are everywhere. They offer vehicle histories, comparative pricing, and feature tools from dealers throughout the country totaling over 40,000 vehicles in inventory. They also provide financing calculators and options to understand what your monthly payment will be. Gone are the days when you sat in a dealership while the sales guy went back and forth with his manager and finance guy to haggle over price with you.[4]

A NEW PERSPECTIVE

Is there any other area of your life where you just go with the status quo? Think about your car. If you're like me, you need it to get from point A to point B. You need it to run well, so you keep it in good shape. If it's having a problem, you know you need to take it to the shop, but you don't go in cold. You do your homework, ask around, and, if you feel that an estimate is too high, you get a second opinion. Nobody wants to get taken advantage of on a car repair. Why should your health be any different? It shouldn't.

Just like your car needs to run, you need your health to be at a certain level to preserve your quality of life. Sometimes you need to check in. Sometimes you might even need a tune-up. You're not at the mercy of your mechanic,

---

4   Arata, Nicole. "10 Top Car-Buying Apps." NerdWallet. September 14, 2017. Accessed September 07, 2018. https://www.nerdwallet.com/blog/loans/top-car-buying-apps/.

so why are you at the mercy of the doctors and insurers? Here's the kicker: you're not. You can find a better deal, a better fit. You can vote with your feet and with your wallet.

If you're like many people, maybe you don't realize you've become passive when it comes to your healthcare. Or, maybe you're like me, and you're mad as hell. Look, it's fine to be mad as hell about the current state of healthcare, but we can do something about it! The following pages offer a course of action—a prescription, if you will— for real results.

YOU'RE NOT ALONE

Just look at the recent headlines made by Amazon, Berkshire, and Chase as they released their intentions to form a nonprofit health entity. Change is coming! They are not going to take it anymore. Why should you?

Medical costs are "like a hungry tapeworm on the American economy."—Warren Buffett[5]

"Since 2000, price, and NOT demand for services or

---

5   Tuttle, Brad. "Warren Buffett, Jeff Bezos, Jamie Dimon: Cheaper Health Care | Money." Time. January 30, 2018. Accessed April 04, 2018. http://time.com/money/5124642/warren-buffett-jeff-bezos-cheaper-health-care-insurance-costs/.

aging of the population, has produced 91 percent of the cost increases in the US healthcare system today."[6]

No one's been talking *with* you about healthcare and insurance all these years; they've been talking *at* you. Not me. I'll be your partner, empowering you every step of the way. If, in the end, you trust yourself to make the best decisions for yourself and your family—and you know the right questions to ask if you encounter a problem—I will have done my job.

Thank you for giving this book a chance to help you take back control of your healthcare. We are going to start you at the beginning: understanding who you are and who you might become health-wise. We are then going to learn what health services cost. Coupled with that information, we will address how you will pay for the health services and what insurance plans would be appropriate for your budget, and known and potential expenses, given the cost of healthcare. We will then talk about maximizing your outcomes with providers using transparency tools to understand their capabilities and how they match your needs, and we'll discuss how to negotiate with those providers to reach the optimum balance between high quality and best cost. Finally, we will talk about how to

---

6 Moses, 3. R., D. H. Matheson, E. R. Dorsey, B. P. George, D. Sadoff, and S. Yoshimura. "The Anatomy of Health Care in the United States." JAMA. November 13, 2013. Accessed April 04, 2018. https://www.ncbi.nlm.nih.gov/pubmed/24219951.

proactively manage your own health through lifestyle choices which don't cost anything!

Buckle up; it's going to be a wild ride.

CHAPTER TWO

WHY WE ARE WHERE WE ARE: THE THIRD-PARTY SYNDROME

Taking control of your healthcare starts by being proactive rather than reactive. As I said earlier, you do have power here; you just need to understand how to use it. And much of that power begins with understanding that no one is going to care more about the level of care you receive, and how much you pay for it, than *you*.

I get it: most people don't understand how healthcare or health insurance works. No one actually *chooses* to be a healthcare consumer—we all simply *are*, regardless of race, creed, color, position, or socioeconomic status. Taking care of your health is simply a human necessity.

Because it is an unplanned necessity, most of us go into the healthcare complex woefully unprepared. That makes us vulnerable to costly undesirable results.

Let's review how we got where we are.

Third-party health payments started in the 1920s with hospitals offering pre-payment plans. What quickly followed was the development of Blue Cross organizations forming with the first employer-based health insurance plan offered to teachers in Dallas, Texas, in 1929. Employer-paid healthcare grew significantly in the Forties and Fifties as a way to offer unions and their members what were relatively inexpensive offerings, rather than conceding to raising their wages. The proliferation of group insurance plans (49.7 percent of the population covered today) led to the direct relationship between providers (hospitals) and the health insurance companies. The Nineties saw the explosion of managed care companies (Health Maintenance Organizations, HMO; and Preferred Provider Organizations, PPO). These health insurance policies managed who you could see, when you could see them, how much it would cost, and what services could be performed—further excluding the consumer from making their own healthcare decisions. Without direct input into the pricing of the services, our healthcare cost awareness diminished and eventually died.

Then, we have the compounding effect of the Affordable Care Act, ACA (Obamacare), which went into effect in January 2014. ACA was passed to combat the sizable number of uninsured Americans and the astronomically rising healthcare service and insurance costs. The positive aspects of ACA include the following: the elimination of preexisting conditions that would allow health insurance companies to deny coverage based on a previously known condition, the standardization of plans offered, the uncapping of annual or lifetime spending limits on insurance plans, and the governmental subsidies based on income to pay for health insurance or be included in Medicaid, i.e., government health insurance for the poor.

Was it effective? On one hand, the number of uninsured Americans was cut in half with approximately twenty million Americans gaining healthcare insurance coverage. No one is turned down for insurance, and you can no longer run out of your insurance with a catastrophic claim. On the other hand, healthcare insurance premiums have continued to skyrocket, access is limited because of the number of carriers not offering coverage in certain areas of the country, and the financial sustainability of the program is questionable.

Here are major implications of the challenges:

- The average 2018 premium increase range for individual insurance offered through the public exchange was 34–38 percent.[7]

- The number of counties with only one individual healthcare insurer is growing.
- Claims over one million dollars have increased 68 percent between 2014 and 2017.[8]
- Over 50 percent of insured individuals are on high-deductible plans.

Whoever said pictures are worth a thousand words knew what they were talking about. Look at these charts from a July 2018 *Wall Street Journal* article titled, "Why Americans Spend So Much on Health Care—in 12 Charts."[9]

7   "NHE-Fact-Sheet." CMS.gov Centers for Medicare & Medicaid Services. February 14, 2018. Accessed April 10, 2018. https://www.cms.gov/research-statistics-data-and-systems/statistics-trends-and-reports/nationalhealthexpenddata/nhe-fact-sheet.html.

8   "2017 Sun Life Stop-Loss Research Report." Sun Life Financial - United States. Accessed August 15, 2018. http://www.sunlife.com/us/News and insights/Insights/2017 Sun Life Stop-Loss research report.

9   Walker, Joseph. "Why Americans Spend So Much on Health Care-In 12 Charts." The Wall Street Journal. July 31, 2018. Accessed August 14, 2018. https://www.wsj.com/articles/why-americans-spend-so-much-on-health-carein-12-charts-1533047243.

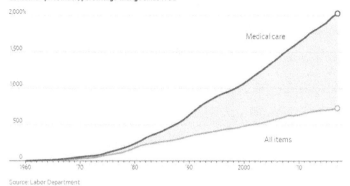

Source: Labor Department

Drug prices have risen the most of the three largest components of health spending since 2000, followed by hospital care and physician services.

Price growth since 2000

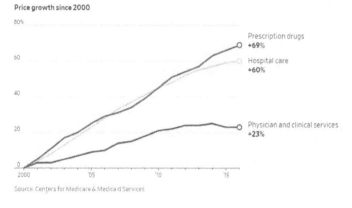

Source: Centers for Medicare & Medicaid Services

In sum, we have more people adequately covered, but prices still continue to rise. Did ACA impact the third-party players rendering and paying for care? It sure did! Insurance companies that predicted their demise if pre-existing conditions were removed without universal coverage have not fared too badly. A look at the stock price returns of what insiders call the BUCAs (Blue Cross

Blue Shield, United Healthcare, Cigna, and Aetna) since 2014–2016 show a 156 percent return vs the S&P at 91 percent.[10] You don't necessarily need to understand the stock market to get the larger picture here: stock prices don't normally go up if you are losing money or even breaking even.

Then, you have the hospitals. With the annual or lifetime caps removed from health insurance plans and twenty million more Americans covered under some form of health insurance, the hospitals have not fared too badly. Just look at the skyline around any city from downtown to the suburbs, and you will see construction cranes. Look closely and see what they are building; more often than not, it's a hospital expansion. Further support is provided by an article in the Cincinnati Enquirer highlighting Children's Hospitals' indigent care (services provided at no cost to those who cannot afford care) before and after the implementation of ACA. Prior to ACA being enacted, Children's Hospitals' indigent care rate was 25 percent. After ACA, it decreased to 10 percent; in addition, after ACA, insurance plans could no longer limit or cap the amount a policy would cover. This new rule essentially gives hospitals the ability to collect more and more. I am not questioning that people, and especially children, ben-

10 Coombs, Bertha. "As Obamacare Twists in Political Winds, Top Insurers Profits Surge Nearly 30 Percent." CNBC. August 06, 2017. Accessed August 15, 2018. https://www.cnbc.com/2017/08/05/top-health-insurers-profit-surge-29-percent-to-6-billion-dollars.html.

efit from an uncapped insurance plan. But where does all that additional money paid to the hospital go? Have hospitals reduced their service charges? Have they launched an entirely privately funded expansion plan?[11] Hospitals deny profiting from ACA by pointing to their declining inpatient occupancy rates but gloss over the shift of their business to outpatient services—which are thriving.

Here's the "third-party" kicker. The *Wall Street Journal* article I discussed earlier mentioned health insurance companies that provide the managed care networks that provide discounts to their insureds must spend 85 percent of every dollar they make on medical expenses for the insured. They can only keep 15 percent for administration, operating costs, and profit. If their actual medical expenses drop, they are required by ACA to return, in a dividend, money to their insureds. Brilliant maneuver by ACA, right? Let's take a closer look: insurers can only keep 15 percent; that's a percent, not a fixed dollar amount. So, as the price of claims increases, insurers get paid more without any additional services or incurred risk. In essence, they make more money. What has happened in the market? We know claims over one million dollars have increased 68 percent from Sun Life's Stop Loss report, cited previously. This report is for employer-paid insurance, so it isn't impacted by the twenty million Americans

11   Bizjournals.com. Accessed August 15, 2018. https://www.bizjournals.com/cincinnati/ news/2017/03/17/first-look-children-s-hospital-reveals-cost.html.

now receiving Medicaid or individually purchased coverage. It's an apple-to-apple of covered members before and after ACA. Maybe that's why insurance carriers' stock prices have gone up so much since ACA.

Now, we have the hospital and insurance negotiators who were traditionally pitted against each other aligned in their goals. Hospitals are receiving more covered individuals and don't have their expenses capped. Insurance carriers make more by law as the prices and number of hospital services go up. Who's working for us?

Effective consumers of any product, especially in this day and age, start out researching. They find out the quality of the product or service they want and the price. They then make an informed decision about which product they will purchase. Think about it: How long would you keep buying your smartphone without knowing the monthly cost, the service area, etc.? Would you just keep paying that bill anyway? No, you wouldn't, but that is how the healthcare industry is set up. Up until now, because of lack of information (transparency) and the third-party system, you—the consumer—didn't know what healthcare costs or how to compare outcomes by provider. It's not a good recipe if you want to have your voice heard and experience cost-effective healthcare.

Other factors impeding our ability to become informed

healthcare consumers are traditional lack of pricing and outcome transparency, what I call insurance lethargy and the doctor mystique. Insurance lethargy describes the collective attitude toward insurance. If you have a health insurance plan these days, one way or the other, you are paying a lot of money in premium guaranteed every month. You then have the privilege to pay more when you actually incur a health expense—i.e., you see a doctor. As a result, when your insurance plan finally begins to cover all expenses at 100 percent, you mentally check out. You think, "I don't care what the services cost, how many are performed, if they are necessary, or if services not provided are on the bill." You simply disengage—and understandably so. You've paid a lot of money to get where you are. Remember this, though: an insurance policy renews every year; every year, the premiums inevitably go up. Why? Because expenses go up.

CASE IN POINT

I work with a CFO who handles the health renewals for his company. One day, he asked me what project I was working on, and I explained I was writing this book to empower individuals to become consumers of healthcare. "Why would anyone care once they hit the 100 percent level of payment from their insurance policy?" he asked. I replied, "What happens every January at your company?" He paused and said, "Health insurance renewal." I then asked what would happen if all his employees fought for the most effective procedures at the best cost all year round. The answer is clear: lower health insurance premiums.

Last but certainly not the least is the "doctor mystique." A friend and noted radiologist at a major Midwestern medical state university put it this way, "Over the past sixty years, medical care has experienced great strides and accomplishments: antibiotics (penicillin), killer-disease-eradicating vaccines (chicken pox, smallpox, polio), and organ transplants (heart, lung, kidney, etc.). Patients have grown to expect a cure for whatever they have and to revere their medical professionals. Challenging courses of treatment and costs with your provider seems counterproductive and disrespectful, but escalating costs and the efficacy of the treatments need to be discussed and reviewed."

He's right.

DON'T LIKE IT? CHANGE IT. HERE'S HOW.

Bob is self-employed and has carried family health insurance his entire life. He doesn't qualify for any of the ACA subsidies to offset premiums. No one in his family has serious or chronic medical conditions. Although his medical insurance premiums never thrilled him, they were manageable. Then came ACA. His premiums rose to $12,000 per year, and his family deductible and out-of-pocket costs increased to over $12,000. Ultimately, that means before healthcare picks up at 100 percent for his entire family, he has to spend $24,000 per year. Sound familiar?

Highlighting and reviewing the whys of where we are will not affect change, but it does give us a roadmap of what we need to address. If you are at the end of your rope with higher premiums and out-of-pocket medical costs every year and concerned that they will break you financially, then you are ready to try something different. That's what I'm hoping for. I'm going to dissect each area that has led us to where we are and provide tools and techniques to help you become an informed, confident consumer of healthcare.

First and foremost, you need to understand you have the right and obligation to get involved. The "third-party" dealings previously illustrated should convince you that you need to look out for your own interests; after all, no one else is. It's your obligation. You also have the right. Most don't know that President Clinton, after failing to pass a precursor to ACA in 1992, proposed a Healthcare Bill of Rights. Although defeated by intense lobbying efforts by both the insurance and hospital industries, features of the bill were included in the ACA. They require insurance companies to provide full disclosure of the plans, policies, and procedures, including what the plans will cover and what they will not. It also requires medical providers to maintain patient privacy; consult and gain consent with treatment, including risks and benefits of treatments and alternative care; and understand cost.

Secondly, you must become a knowledgeable, confident consumer of the whole continuum: health insurance, healthcare service, and your own health status. To be successful, you need to develop your own goals and objectives by doing the following:

- Understanding your current health status and family health histories
- Understanding your conditions or potential condition costs
- Understanding your financial resources
- Selecting insurance policies that cover those requirements
- Selecting the best cost-effective medical providers aligned with your needs
- Communicating effectively with your providers regarding treatment plans and cost
- Proactively managing your health to avoid the need for costly healthcare services

Luckily, this isn't 1992. There are transparency tools available to assist with your research. Knowledge is power! Whether or not the medical community is ready for it, pricing and quality outcome reporting is becoming available to you. Furthermore, you are directly paying your providers more and more each year—a fact that, alone, entitles you to a voice. Finally, the power of social media to move markets and break decades' worth of habits and barriers has morphed over the past few short years. (Think of the #MeToo movement.)

Do you think this is all hyperbole and soapbox preaching? Let me share two examples to prove it's not.

Jeff took a blood thinner that cost $380/month. Jeff had a $5,000 high-deductible plan, so every dollar spent up to $5,000 was out of his pocket. The annual charges of the drug were only $4,560, which was below the $5,000 deductible. What that means is the insurance did not pay for any of the drug cost; he paid 100 percent. Jeff inquired with his doctor about lower-cost alternatives and was told that, for his situation, the expensive blood thinner was the best option. Still not satisfied, he researched the drug industry and found a manufacturer's program that reduced his cost to $10/month because he was paying for the drug. That's a $4,440 annual savings with one phone call.

A few years ago, a subsidiary of Mylan, a large pharmaceutical company, bought the EpiPen. It is a decade's old serum—epinephrine or adrenaline—delivered in a decade's old delivery system used to counteract difficulty breathing due to severe allergic reactions. Prices for a pen were $50–$70. Their marketing department saw a way to tag along with the government's requirement that all public schools carry a food-borne allergy antidote: without changing anything the EpiPen already fit that mold. By selling to the government-funded public schools their sales increased, and so did their pricing—eventually topping out at $600 per pen. Furthermore, Mylan claimed the drug lost its potency after a year and only sold the pens in two-packs. What was a fifty-million-dollar business became close to one-billion-dollar business, all with a solution that had been around since 1970.[12]

Mothers and fathers with higher deductible insurance plans received quite a cost jolt as the price of the EpiPen jumped. They took to the internet reaching for help. Eventually, the buzz grew loud enough for politicians on political campaigns (Hillary Clinton) and others to put pressure on the company. The CEO was summoned to testify before Congress. Such pressure lead Mylan to reduce the cost and also accelerated other alternatives to the market within two years—one of which was provided

12 Ramsey, Lydia. "The Strange History of the EpiPen, the Device Developed by the Military That Turned into a Billion-dollar Business and Now Faces Generic Competition between Mylan and Teva." Business Insider. August 17, 2018. Accessed September 06, 2018. https:// www.businessinsider.com/the-history-of-the-epipen-and-epinephrine-2016-8.

by Walgreens and was priced closer to Mylan's original amount.[13]

Parents experiencing sticker shock reacted like any consumer would: they made themselves known, and the market responded. Would they have made themselves known if they hadn't been paying for it?

These two examples highlight multiple levels of knowledge, communication, negotiation, and perseverance. This book will address each area, citing examples, tools, and techniques that you can adopt to become a better consumer. Note, though, that shifting paradigms and years of fixed behavior doesn't happen overnight; it requires proactive effort and practice to become proficient and the confidence to do so. There's no Magic 8 Ball that provides neatly packaged answers to your questions and situations. There's not one approach or style that is guaranteed to work. You will develop your own approach and style that fits your needs, and you will need to learn it and practice it.

In his book *Outliers*, Malcolm Gladwell asserted that 10,000 hours of practice defines the exceptional from the ordinary. Gladwell cited a quote from John Lennon on

13   Edwards, Haley Sweetland. "EpiPen Cost: Hillary Clinton Proposes Fix to Rising Prices." *Time*. September 02, 2016. Accessed September 07, 2018. http://time.com/4477455/epipen-hillary-clinton/.

one of the factors of the Beatles' success. Lennon recalled when they fine-tuned their skills (referencing their stint in Hamburg, Germany, where they played seven days a week), that they had to play hours on end, that every song lasted for twenty minutes and had twenty solos and there was nobody to cover for them.[14] I'm sure the Beatles had many a misstep in those early sessions, but they played through and became better for it—and so will you. Armed with your new goals, newfound knowledge, and the benefits of practice, you will gain the confidence to effectively enhance your healthcare outcomes.

Let's get started defining who you are health-wise.

14   "Why the Beatles Were so Good: They Practiced!" The Wayward Journey. February 19, 2014. Accessed August 15, 2018. https://waywardjourney.com/2014/02/19/why-the-beatles-were-so-good-they-practiced/.

PART I

PREPARING TO PRACTICE: KNOW YOURSELF AND YOUR RISK

CHAPTER THREE

WHO AM I?

I read an Aetna success story about a man named John who was two steps from a heart attack. In 2010, he took a Health Risk Assessment through his employer. His cholesterol and blood pressure were both off the charts. The news of his high cholesterol was particularly alarming, since he'd been on medication for it the previous two years. He couldn't argue with the facts: he was forty-seven years old, 300 pounds, and had had two knee surgeries because of his weight. Armed with the results from the Health Risk Assessment, he knew he needed to change. He got a health coach who helped him create a game plan to lose some weight. Eventually, he lost 125 pounds. He's even off cholesterol medicine now.[15] In short, he changed his life. John's story is not unique.

---

15 "Two Steps from a Heart Attack." Eye Movement Desensitization and Reprocessing (EMDR) Therapy - Medical Clinical Policy Bulletins | Aetna. Accessed September 07, 2018. https://www. aetna.com/individuals-families/member-success-stories/big-john-rowgo-loses-weight.html.

There are many stories out there of people like John—people who see a health problem in their life and take steps to fix it. The percentage who actually follow through, though, is small—in my experience, it's about 6 percent. You need something personal to motivate you. There has to be a catalyst that kicks you in the rear end. For John, he should've realized something was wrong when he had those two knee surgeries because of his weight. He knew he wasn't feeling his best. It wasn't until the report told him, "Be ready. You're a walking heart attack," that something clicked in him.

Don't wait for a report to tell you you're dying to take control of your health. Start your healthcare journey earlier than you think you should. It will be uncomfortable, and you'll encounter a lot of questions. For example, you know you need health insurance, but how much should you get and why? What will it cost? What should it cover? When selecting a doctor or hospital, which ones are experts in the areas I need addressed? How much do they charge? What are their patient outcomes after treatment? In order to answer those questions, you must know who you are first. You do this by taking a look at what your needs are, what your resources are, then going to the market and seeing who matches them.

FIRST THINGS FIRST

Knowing your needs as a healthcare consumer comes down to defining who you are, identifying your risks, and identifying your costs. You start with defining who you are because without that understanding, you won't know what to buy. You could over-buy or under-buy insurance, and both of those are bad decisions.

Like any other problem-solving technique, we'll approach taking back control of your healthcare by breaking the problem into components and solving them one at a time.

1. Develop your objective or identify the problem.
2. Conduct research on the subject.
3. Plot out a game plan.
4. Enact the plan.

In short, first you'll become familiar with who you are as a healthcare consumer. Then, you'll become knowledgeable about your options. Finally, you'll become comfortable putting your insight into action!

IT STARTS WITH A HEALTH RISK ASSESSMENT

What John did by taking that Health Risk Assessment was smart, even if he waited too long to do it. This assessment has a standard set of questions that helps develop your health profile. It assesses your health status, estimates your level of health risk, and provides feedback to guide your behaviors. Information collected includes your demographic information (age and sex), lifestyle information (alcohol intake, exercise habits, whether or not you smoke, etc.), personal and family medical history, physiological data (weight, height, blood pressure, etc.), and your attitudes and willingness to change your behavior in order to improve your health. The HRA compiles and analyzes your information and produces your health risk profile. Your profile ranks your health in seven key health areas: heart, cancer, diabetes, obesity, nutrition, fitness, and mental and emotional health through color-coding, graphs, icons, and a number-based scoring system that tells you if you are doing well, need to be cautious, or need to take immediate action. It recommends key ways to improve your scores and health. The report is printable so that it can be exchanged with your physician.[16]

16   Wellsource. (2018). *Employee and Member Health Risk Assessments | HRA Company.* [online]
      Available at: https://www.wellsource.com/products/health-assessments/wellsuite-iv-health-
      risk-assessment-for-the-workforce-us/ [Accessed 22 Oct. 2018].

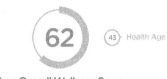

Your Overall Wellness Score

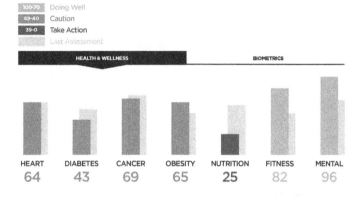

How can you get your own health risk profile? About 33 percent of employers offer these HRAs (Health Risk Assessments) through their employee health plan. For companies with over 200 employees, that number goes up to 51 percent. Many of them even have an app you can use to securely give and receive information for your health risk profile. Medicare and Medicaid both offer HRAs as well, as do some hospitals. Check with your local hospital to see if they have one.

Not too long ago, you had to do these HRAs on paper. Now, you can complete them on your phone through an app or on your computer through a website. It's so easy that there's no excuse not to do it, especially because much of the information required can be gathered at a basic physical (which is 100 percent covered if you have a plan under the ACA). Be sure the information you're entering is recent—that is, taken within a six-month window, especially for test results. Why is this so important? Understanding your basic health status is the first step in identifying what your objectives need to be. Your objectives clarify and direct you to which tools and options are right for you. A health risk profile is a perfect way to discover what type of insurance and providers you should be pursuing.

COMPILING YOUR HEALTH RECORD

After completing an HRA, you need to compile all your medical history to complete your total health profile. At first, it will feel laborious. It's like setting up Quicken, the personal budgeting software, for the first time, or transferring all of your files to a new computer—not a joyous experience, but you've got to do it! It entails gathering all of your health records, including documentation of conditions, biometrics, physicals, immunizations, surgeries, imaging, diagnostic test results, and medications. It should include a thorough understanding of family conditions. Interview your parents about your family health history. If you discover a family history of a genetic condition, after consulting with your doctor, you want to weigh the pros and cons of genetic testing to determine if you are at risk of developing the condition. For example, certain types of tests may be useful in identifying your risk of certain types of colorectal cancer.

So, how do you access your information? With the exception of your family history, all of your data is moving to electronic data interchange (EDI) and storage, so you can call your hospital, doctor, or specialist and ask to download your records (lab work, diagnostic imaging, doctor's notes). If you are unable to pursue the electronic route, paper records are just as effective. At the very least, keep a list of doctors or hospitals where you have received or are receiving care, what conditions you have been or are being treated for, and what medications you are taking and for what purpose.

These records complete your in-depth health profile. Having full access to your records, electronically or via hard copy, will help you communicate effectively with your doctor in an efficient manner. That way, they can more accurately assess your conditions and prescribe effective courses of treatment.

WHAT'S NEXT? PERSONAL TECHNOLOGY

Apple, Google, Fitbit, and others are working on electronically integrating the consumer with their providers and medical information. Companies in Silicon Valley are realizing that healthcare is one-sixth of the US economy, and they want their piece of it. They are developing ways to transfer medical records between all vested participants, as well as monitoring patients' conditions remotely 24/7. The potential outcome enhancements and cost-reduction benefits are three-fold: more accurate diagnosis, a reduction in duplicate testing, and increased treatment compliance.

This isn't science fiction; it's reality. Even now, if you have an iPhone, check the home screen for the white box with the red heart. You have a health record app built-in! Try it out.

Note: The major concerns about recording personal private health information on the vast web have been addressed. Privacy protections were outlined in the Health Insurance Portability and Accountability Act (HIPAA 1996). You sign a HIPAA form every time you go to the doctor's office. And, the ACA (2010) required all medical providers to transmit patient data electronically, while eliminating preexisting condition exclusions from health insurance. The biggest prior fear was that insurance carriers would find out about your health status and decline coverage or upcharge you. Not anymore!

Now that you have an idea of who you are from a health status, let's look at the cost of healthcare by conditions.

CHAPTER FOUR

WHAT ARE THE ACTUAL COSTS OF HEALTHCARE?

The average lifetime costs of healthcare for an American woman are $361,200 and $268,000 for a man.[17] This is partly due to the fact that women live longer than men and also have to incur the costs of childbirth. All in all, healthcare costs amount to an average of $10,348 per person per year (in 2016). This works out to 17.9 percent of the country's GDP.

There's one key commonality: nobody truly knows how much healthcare *actually* costs. That changes today—I'm going to help you find ways to uncover what the costs are.

---

17 Alemayehu, Berhanu, and Kenneth E. Warner. Advances in Pediatrics. June 2004. Accessed August 15, 2018. https://www.ncbi.nlm.nih.gov/pmc/articles/PMC1361028/.

How do those national averages translate to you, the consumer, when you're in the doctor's office, ER, or hospital and are confronting the cost of your care and how you're going to pay for it? What can you expect to find? Most people have no idea what their healthcare services actually cost.

WHAT COSTS WILL YOU FACE?

After you complete your Health Risk Assessment, you'll have a better idea of who you are health-wise. You'll know what ailments might be coming your way or if you can expect to be healthy as a rose. Then what do you do? Here I'll run through some of the most common healthcare charges you'll encounter, all of which vary depending on the severity of the issue and your geography. Depending on your health, you can use these charges to determine how you'll approach paying for conditions you have or are prone to have.[18]

COMMON HEALTHCARE COSTS

- Male physical exam: $200–$240
- Female physical exam, age eighteen to forty: $185–$240
- Female physical exam, over forty: $280–$330

---

18   About Guroo.com | Health Care Cost Institute (HCCI)." Health Care Cost Institute. Accessed August 15, 2018. http://www.healthcostinstitute.org/about-hcci/about-guroo/.

- Child physical exam: $160-$180
- Adult doctor's visit (for common ailments): $130-$180
- Child doctor's visit: $114-$160
- Adult emergency room (not including tests): $580-$700
- Child emergency room (not including tests): $510-$635
- Allergy study: $220-$370
- Electrocardiogram: $40-$100
- Echocardiogram: $75-$225
- Pulmonary study: $25-$100
- Sleep study: $100-$600
- Blood count test: $5-$20
- Urinalysis test: $5-$15
- Hematology: $15-$30
- Colonoscopy: $750-$950
- Cardiac catheterization: $500-$2,500
- MRI: $500-$1,300
- CAT scan: $400-$700
- Pregnancy, vaginal delivery: $9,800-$11,000
- Pregnancy, C-section delivery: $11,500-$12,700
- Broken arm: $180
- X-ray: $65
- Diabetic visits (two or three): $318
- Dermatologist visit: $145
- Chiropractic visits (series of six): $200
- Physical therapist visits for back pain (series of six): $533

- Vertebrae fusion: $70,000

Get ready for some shock therapy; we're moving into the costs associated with more catastrophic situations.[19]

- Malignant neoplasm (general cancer): $139,843
- Leukemia: $229,568
- Chronic end-stage renal disease: $227,546
- Issues related to short gestation (premature births): $235,245
- Transplants: $242,578
- Congestive heart failure: $181,320
- Cerebrovascular diseases (blood clots, strokes): $129,024
- Pulmonary collapse: $122,721
- Septicemia: $173,912

If you suffer a catastrophic event, the cost for that occurrence might not be the only fees you'll incur as a result. Take Septicemia, for example, which are bacterial infections that are becoming more of an issue as they gain resistance to antibiotics. If you go in for a transplant, for example, and wind up an infection that leads to septice-

---

19 "2017 Sun Life Stop-Loss Research Report." Sun Life Financial - United States. Accessed August 15, 2018. http://www.sunlife.com/us/News and insights/Insights/2017 Sun Life Stop-Loss research report.

mia on top of it, that's $173,912 on top of the $242,578 for the transplant. Do you see how costs can compound? You haven't seen anything yet.

CATASTROPHIC EVENT HIGH-END COSTS

I've shared the average costs of catastrophic events. Now, let's take a look at the high-end costs for those same illnesses, according to Sun Life.[20] Buckle up.

- Malignant neoplasm: $3.2 million
- Leukemia: $2.3 million
- Chronic end-stage renal disease: $3 million
- Genital issues at birth: $2.8 million
- Issues related to short gestation: $4 million
- Transplants: $2.2 million
- Congestive heart failure: $3.8 million
- Cerebrovascular diseases (blood clots, strokes): $3.1 million
- Pulmonary collapse: $1.7 million
- Septicemia: $2.7 million

Disturbing, isn't it? Here's more disturbing news about these mega-claims in the US as we pointed out earlier: instances of one-million-dollar claims nearly doubled

---

20 "Press Releases." Sun Life Financial - United States. Accessed August 15, 2018. http://www. sunlife.com/us/News and insights/Press releases/2016/Top Ten Catastrophic Claims Conditions report explores costliest medical conditions and emerging trends

between 2016 and 2017, and multi-million-dollar claims have increased 68 percent. How do you financially protect yourself?

The price estimates were gathered from Sun Life Insurance Company's 2017 annual large claim report and accessing the transparency tool Guroo. We will explore in greater detail the burgeoning medical transparency tools available to you, the consumer, in chapter 6.

CHAPTER FIVE

MANAGING THE RISK

Richard, a heating and cooling mechanic, was complaining about Obamacare. About the rising costs. About the system being rigged against people like him. About maybe just abstaining from insurance completely the next time enrollment came around. Then, I saw it—the ring on his finger.

"So, are you married?" I asked.

"Yes," he said.

"Do you have kids? Do you have a house? A car?" I asked.

"Yep."

"And do you insure the house and the cars?"

"Yes, of course."

"Why?" I asked.

"Well, if my house burns down, I've got to replace it. I've got to pay to rebuild it. If I wreck my car, I need to get a new one."

"Perfect," I said. "What happens if you get sick and you don't have insurance, or you're stuck with insurance that isn't going to cover what you need it to?"

"Well," he said, "I don't know. We'll just take care of it, I guess."

"Look," I told him. "If you get stuck with a catastrophic $200,000 healthcare bill and you're not properly insured, you realize the hospital can take your house, right? It's an asset. Insuring yourself is no different than insuring your house, and it's more important in the long run."

He looked at me for a long time and said, "Nobody's ever explained it to me like that before."

CONDUCT YOUR FINANCIAL RISK ASSESSMENT

Based on your known and potential risks and how much you could be spending on health conditions, my guess is that no one reading this book can afford or would want to afford the catastrophic claims, and no one with chronic conditions would want to pay the full amounts previously illustrated. Certainly, Richard would have reached a different conclusion on his own after reading the first chapters. If you're a young male with no known personal or family health conditions, maybe you are not concerned—but should you be? How are we going to manage the risk?

There are three ways to manage (transfer) risk: self-insure, avoidance, or insure. Self-insuring is not a reasonable option given the cost of catastrophic claims shown earlier. Avoiding risk would mean not getting sick, which is not as ridiculous as it sounds and a concept we will explore in lifestyle management (although not a financially prudent option). That leaves transferring the risk: insurance.

Let's talk about insurance and risk. Google's definition of insurance reads, "a practice or arrangement by which a company or government agency provides a guarantee of compensation for specified loss, damage, illness, or death in return for payment of a premium." That's where we are. Our analysis has determined we need to pay a premium to transfer or offset potential loss due to illness or unforeseen accident, but what's the right amount of insurance we need to buy?

My consulting practice analyzed whether companies should self-insure or insure their employee benefit healthcare programs. We adhered to the rule that you do not insure what is predictable and affordable within your own means. Otherwise, you are overpaying for the risk transfer. We have already illustrated health insurance companies are doing exceptionally well by being paid 15 percent in addition to actual medical costs. Who pays the health insurance companies the premiums? YOU DO! Why, then, would you pay the insurance company an extra 15 percent on items that are predictable and you can afford to pay? You shouldn't. We will explore creative ways and tax-incented avenues to help pay for predictable items in later sections.

Look at it this way: most of us buy car insurance to protect us from costs arising from accidents—damages and liability, occurrences we cannot predict nor afford. What do you think the cost of those insurance policies would be if covered items included gas, new tires, oil changes, tune ups, and the like? Get my point?

HEALTH INSURANCE PURCHASING CHECKLIST

Let's delve into the work you have done so far and build your health insurance calculator decision tool. Before I inundate you with the myriad medical insurance plan types on the market and their various nuances, I want to establish a checklist to determine which plans meet your needs. Medical insurance policies are sold for twelve-month periods of time and thus focus on the next twelve months of anticipated medical expenses.

The checklist introduces new concepts and terms that will be forthcoming. It will be appropriate for you to review this checklist after completing those chapters.

STEP ONE

Consult your recently created personal health record and history and determine your known or anticipated medical expenses for the coming year. The list needs to include physician office visits, prescriptions, diagnostic and lab work, and medical procedures.

STEP TWO

Identify the plans available to you, the amount of coverage they offer, and the amount of upfront dollars you will need to pay. The terms you will need to familiarize yourself with are premiums, deductibles, copays, and out-of-pocket charges.

PREMIUMS, COPAYS, DEDUCTIBLES, AND COINSURANCE

These cost components—premiums, copays, deductibles, coinsurance, and out-of-pocket maximums—are common to almost all plans. They determine how much you will pay for health insurance and are the health insurance plans' differentiating features. They are the features you will have to consider each year when you elect health insurance. Premiums are a guaranteed monthly expense, but these items only come into play when you utilize healthcare. Plans offer a range of each of the above. That is why we've spent time understanding who you are, what expenses you might have next year, and what your health status is long term. That work will direct you to the appropriate plan for you.

Premium: The premium is the amount of money that an individual or business must pay for an insurance policy. The insurance premium is income for the insurance company, once it is earned, and also represents a liability in that the insurer must provide coverage for claims being made against the policy.

Copay: Your copay is a predetermined rate you pay for healthcare services at the time of care. For example, you may have a $25 copay every time you see your primary care physician, a $10 copay for each monthly medication, and a $250 copay for an emergency room visit.

Deductible: The deductible is how much you pay before your health insurance starts to cover a larger portion of your bills. In general, if you have a $1,000 deductible, you must pay $1,000 for your own care out-of-pocket before your insurer starts covering a higher portion of costs. The deductible resets yearly.

Coinsurance: Coinsurance is a percentage of a medical charge that you pay, with the rest paid by your health insurance plan after your deductible has been met. For example, if you have a 20 percent coinsurance, you pay 20 percent of each medical bill, and your health insurance will cover 80 percent.

Out-of-pocket maximum: The most you could have to pay in one year, out of-pocket, for your healthcare before your insurance covers 100 percent of the bill. The out-of-pocket maximum for any accredited ACA plan is $7,900 for a single plan and $15,800 for a family plan; or $6,750 for a single and $13,500 for a family for a type of plan called a Health Savings Account (HSA)-compatible High-Deductible Plan (HDHP) (2019).

NOTE: Plans may offer different levels of benefits for in- and out-of-network benefits.

STEP THREE

Compare your anticipated medical expenses plus the premiums and out-of-pocket costs of each and every health plan available to you. Don't automatically exclude any, even those with a high deductible. Do the math. Which plan costs you the least in total?

STEP FOUR

Compare the total out-of-pocket costs of each plan versus your cash flow (how much you can afford monthly). Ask yourself if you can handle your healthcare costs in one payment or, if not, how much you can afford monthly. For example, can your pocketbook sustain $694 in monthly costs, or $8,365 annually? Be realistic.

TIP

Many employer enrollment programs provide healthcare calculators for you, or you can search the web for some. Check out MVPHealthCare.com, a platform that sells high-deductible plans to employers but has a plan calculator available on their website. You can also try the Kaiser Family Foundation.

STEP FIVE

Determine what hospitals and doctors are covered

as "in-network or network" doctors. Are your current doctors "in-network"? If not, and you were to see a non-networked provider, your copay, deductible, coinsurance, and out-of-pocket maximums will generally double, at which point you will have to decide if that doctor/provider warrants the higher costs. If so, revisit the plans in which they are networked providers.

TIP

If you don't have a doctor and are looking to establish a relationship, make sure the doctors in the network are taking new patients. Ask the carrier or call the doctor directly.

STEP SIX

Understand what services are covered and which are not. Note that it's more efficient to study the exclusion section of the policy. If it is not in the material you have been presented with, ask for a copy of the policy (Summary Plan Description). In addition, if you are on prescription medicine, make sure your meds are covered. Ask for a list of covered drugs. You are entitled to this information.

STEP SEVEN

Ask for and study all tax deferring or saving mechanisms available (premium-only plans, flexible spending accounts, health reimbursement accounts, and health savings accounts are all detailed in chapter 7).

After completing the checklist, you should have a clear path to what is the most cost-effective plan that meets your specific needs. Remember, don't overinsure by selecting the plan with the lowest out-of-pocket features, as it will have the highest premium. Premium is a guaranteed monthly payment and nonrefundable. Deductibles, copays, coinsurance, and maximum out-of-pocket expenses are variable and only assessed when medical expenses are incurred. In future chapters, we will be attacking how to reduce those medical costs.

If you have no claims, you will incur no additional cost other than the premium. If you exceed the maximum out-of-pocket costs, then you stop paying, and the plan pays 100 percent. The high-deductible plan will guarantee the lowest premium and potentially allow you to adopt a tax-deferred saving account. For those with situations in between the two aforementioned examples, completing the checklist is essential to determining which plans will work best for you.

CASE STUDY

Sam, a software engineer with a computer software management company, was presented with the following plans at his company's open enrollment period, both of which increased his family's deductibles and out-of-pocket costs.

HIGH Plan Benefit Summary

GENERAL PLAN INFORMATION	IN-NETWORK BENEFITS
Annual Deductible/Family	$5,000
Coinsurance (Who Pays)	75% Plan; 25% You
Office Visit/Exam	$30 copay
Outpatient Specialist Visit	$60 copay
Annual Out-of-Pocket Limit/Family	$10,000
Lifetime Plan Maximum	Unlimited

INPATIENT HOSPITAL SERVICES

Inpatient Hospitalization	You pay 25% after deductible
Semi-Private Room & Board	You pay 25% after deductible
(Including Services and Supplies)	

EMERGENCY SERVICES

Emergency Room	You pay 25% after deductible

MENTAL HEALTH BENEFITS

Inpatient Care	You pay 25% after deductible
Outpatient Care	You pay 25% after deductible

ALCOHOL ABUSE

Inpatient Care

Inpatient Hospitalization	You pay 25% after deductible

Outpatient Care

Outpatient Services	You pay 25% after deductible

GENERAL PLAN INFORMATION	IN-NETWORK BENEFITS

SUBSTANCE ABUSE

Inpatient Care

Inpatient Hospitalization	You pay 25% after deductible

Outpatient Care

Outpatient Services	You pay 25% after deductible

PRESCRIPTION DRUG BENEFITS

Prescription Drug Deductible	N/A
Generic	$10 copay
Brand (Formulary/Preferred)	$35 copay
Brand (Non-Formulary/Non-Preferred)	$50 copay
Number of Days' Supply	31 days

OTHER SERVICES AND SUPPLIES

Chiropractic Services	You pay 25% after deductible

Annual Premium for Family Coverage	$12,109
Out-of-Pocket Family Cost	$10,000
Possible Cost with High Claim	$22,109

The above information is intended as a benefit summary only. It does not include all of the benefit provisions, limitations, and qualifications. If this information conflicts in any way with the contract, the contract will prevail.

VALUE Plan Benefit Summary

GENERAL PLAN INFORMATION	IN-NETWORK BENEFITS
Annual Deductible/Family	$6,000
Coinsurance (Who Pays)	80% Plan; 20% You
Office Visit/Exam	0
Outpatient Specialist Visit	$100
Annual Out-of-Pocket Limit/Family	$13,000
Lifetime Plan Maximum	Unlimited

INPATIENT HOSPITAL SERVICES

Inpatient Hospitalization	You pay 20% after deductible
Semi-Private Room & Board	You pay 20% after deductible
(Including Services and Supplies)	

EMERGENCY SERVICES

Emergency Room	You pay 20% after deductible

MENTAL HEALTH BENEFITS

Inpatient Care	You pay 20% after deductible
Outpatient Care	You pay 20% after deductible

ALCOHOL ABUSE

Inpatient Care

Inpatient Hospitalization	You pay 20% after deductible

Outpatient Care

Outpatient Services	You pay 20% after deductible

SUBSTANCE ABUSE

Inpatient Care

Inpatient Hospitalization   You pay 20% after deductible

Outpatient Care

Outpatient Services   You pay 20% after deductible

PRESCRIPTION DRUG BENEFITS

Prescription Drug Deductible $250

Generic   0

Brand (Formulary/Preferred) $50 copay

Brand (Non-Formulary/Non-Preferred) $100 copay

Specialty $250 copay

Number of Days' Supply   31 days

OTHER SERVICES AND SUPPLIES

Chiropractic Services   You pay 20% after deductible

Annual Premium for Family Coverage $8,752

Out-of-Pocket Family Cost $13,000

Possible Cost with High Claim $21,752

The above information is intended as a benefit summary only. It does not include all of the benefit provisions, limitations, and qualifications. If this information conflicts in any way with the contract, the contract will prevail.

HDHP Plan Benefit Summary

GENERAL PLAN INFORMATION	IN-NETWORK BENEFITS
Annual Deductible/Family	$7,000
Coinsurance (Who Pays)	80% Plan; 20% You
Office Visit/Exam	You pay $30 after deductible
Outpatient Specialist Visit	You pay $60 after deductible
Annual Out-of-Pocket Limit/Family	$12,700
Lifetime Plan Maximum	Unlimited

INPATIENT HOSPITAL SERVICES

Inpatient Hospitalization	You pay 20% after deductible
Semi-Private Room & Board	You pay 20% after deductible
(Including Services and Supplies)	

EMERGENCY SERVICES

Emergency Room	You pay 20% after deductible

MENTAL HEALTH BENEFITS

Inpatient Care	You pay 20% after deductible
Outpatient Care	You pay 20% after deductible

ALCOHOL ABUSE

Inpatient Care

Inpatient Hospitalization	You pay 20% after deductible

Outpatient Care

Outpatient Services	You pay 20% after deductible

SUBSTANCE ABUSE

Inpatient Care

Inpatient Hospitalization	You pay 20% after deductible

Outpatient Care

Outpatient Services	You pay 20% after deductible

PRESCRIPTION DRUG BENEFITS

Prescription Drug Deductible	Must meet plan deductible, then:
Generic	$10 copay
Brand (Formulary/Preferred)	$35 copay
Brand (Non-Formulary/Non-Preferred)	$60 copay
Number of Days' Supply	31 days

OTHER SERVICES AND SUPPLIES

Chiropractic Services	You pay 20% after deductible

Annual Premium for Family Coverage	$7,815
Out-of-Pocket Family Cost	$12,700
Possible Cost with High Claim	$20,515

The above information is intended as a benefit summary only. It does not include all of the benefit provisions, limitations, and qualifications. If this information conflicts in any way with the contract, the contract will prevail.

Sam's wife was pregnant, and his son had an existing health condition. He knew he was facing significant healthcare expenditures from both of over $13,000. He assumed the plan with the lowest deductible was "best." Smart, right? Not exactly: Sam's total cost (premium plus maximum out-of-pocket) is actually less for the highest deductible plan. Were he to have applied his known future expenses to the apparent higher out-of-pocket cost programs and compared premiums of all plans, he would have found that the higher out-of-pocket cost plans netted him over $2,500 of savings for that year—money that I'm sure he could have used elsewhere given the events his family faced. Instead, he let inertia and the upfront fear of what appeared to be more out-of-pocket money incorrectly influence his decision, and it cost him! Don't let that happen to you.

TIP

When it comes to your healthcare, remember this rule: remove emotion; do the math!

CHAPTER SIX

TRANSPARENCY: THE CATALYST FOR YOUR HEALTHCARE REVOLUTION

I have a dear friend who's as close to a family member as a friend can get. He knows I'm writing this book, and, like any good friend, he keeps quizzing me about it. Why should anyone care about what I have to say? He says he simply doesn't understand; if your costs are covered 100 percent after you hit your out-of-pocket maximum, why bother writing a book about it? Why do I do it?

The answer is two-pronged—partly from the financial side, and partly from the quality of life side. The common denominator between them, though, is that it comes down to maximizing your coverage and experience when it comes to insurance.

Let's start with finances: if you get service from a doctor and don't inquire about the course of treatment, the appropriateness of the treatment, and the cost, you'll more than likely have a less than optimal experience. Physicians and hospitals are in BUSINESS. One of their goals is to grow their business as profitably as they can. If you're a passive healthcare consumer, the number of tests, where the tests are performed, and who performs them will affect the financial outcome of your treatment—it'll cost you more!

Now, consider if everyone else with that same policy takes the same approach; they simply keep paying whatever the bill says and, while they may grumble, they don't give it a second thought. What, then, are those expenses going to do? They'll go up. If those expenses go up, the insurance company's expenses go up. What is the insurance company (that's in business like the hospitals and physicians) going to do to your premiums? They are going to go up, too. And this dynamic does not change if you're on your employer's sponsored health plan, buying from the public exchange, or buying insurance directly. As we have discussed, there's no incentive for providers or insurance companies to change if they're not challenged.

They both make more money as the costs go up and are, in effect, negotiating with each other over their goals versus yours. I know the process of learning the ins and outs of the industry can be painful and time consuming, but the benefits are long term.

The other side of the equation is life quality. It seems obvious that you'd want the best doctors, right? Why wouldn't you? Yet, in our society, we haven't adopted the mentality that we should scrutinize doctors the same way we would any other service provider, as they're all not created equal. What do you call the person who finished last in his graduating medical school class? You got it: still a doctor.

To overcome this hurdle, we must start insisting on transparency by any means available to us, and that includes referrals. Referrals can come from anybody close to us, such as friends, other doctors, and even the carriers themselves. Use any tool at your disposal in order to find the best doctor for you. If you do, you'll have a better outcome, which means you save money in the long run and have a better quality of life.

By allowing the status quo to continue—which means not questioning our doctors and paying whatever they tell us to—we are all complicit. It's the equivalent to many well-known actors saying they didn't know about sexual abuse in the entertainment industry. They might have noticed things going on around them, and they didn't think they were right, but they didn't say anything. Now, there are a slew of people coming forward via the #metoo movement. They're calling out the industry and demanding change. It's a revolution.

At the end of the day, when my friend asks me why I'm writing my book, I tell him it's because I can make a difference—and so can you. You can change the definition of an industry, even if it's something as big as healthcare or entertainment. Doing the same thing over and over and expecting a different outcome hasn't worked, so why not try something new? If you choose to try, you'll now be in some good company—Warren Buffet, Jeff Bezos, and Jamie Dimon!

How do you tackle two giant industries representing one-sixth of the economy?

Information! Information will lead to knowledge. As Sir Francis Bacon stated, "Knowledge is power."

Chapter 4 illustrated a range of services and their associated costs to familiarize you with what expenses you might have to pay for conditions you have or may have. What we're going to do now is show you the mark ups on some of those services versus the cost and the range of prices for the same service.

A quick look at information out there on hospital markups provides some staggering numbers. According to a report from John Hopkins University, on average, hospitals mark up their cost 4.32 times and, in some cases, over six times. That's right—for a service that costs them $100, they are charging you between $432-$600. The study also found that "certain types of hospitals had higher markups. In government-run hospitals, the ratio was 3.47; in nonprofit hospitals, 3.79; and in for-profit hospitals, 6.31. System-affiliated hospitals had an average ratio of 4.76, versus 3.54 for independent hospitals, and hospitals with regional market power had an average ratio of 4.56, versus 4.16 for hospitals that lacked such clout—supporting the researchers' finding that hospitals that can mark up prices will do so."[21]

This can also be found in medicines within hospitals. Hospitals mark up medicines an average 500 percent of their cost—and have a markup of 250 percent even after negotiations with insurance carriers.[22]

The confusion does not stop there. HCCI's 2015 report, "National Chartbook on Health Care Prices" found that

---

21 Ercolano, Patrick. "Study: Hospitals charge more than 20 times cost on some procedures to maximize revenue." The Hub. September 08, 2016. Accessed April 19, 2018. https://hub.jhu.edu/2016/09/08/hospital-markups-price-gouging/.

22 Zirkelbach, Robert. "How Much Are Hospitals Marking up the Price of Medicines? The Answer May Surprise You." The Catalyst - A PhRMA Blog. Accessed April 19, 2018. https://catalyst.phrma.org/how-much-are-hospitals-marking-up-the-price-of-medicines-the-answer-may-surprise-you.

there is a wide range of prices for the same services at different hospitals. Prices vary by state and within states as well.[23]

AN EXAMPLE OF PRICING IN DIFFERENT LOCATIONS

According to that same report, the average price for a knee replacement in Tucson, Arizona, is $21,976, about $38,000 less than it would be in Sacramento, California. If a Sacramento knee replacement patient doesn't want to drive the 871 miles to Tucson, he or she could drive south to Riverside, California, and pay $27,000 less. In Florida, the surgery costs $17,000 less in Miami than it does 180 miles north in Palm Bay. "The research compared average state vs. national pricing for 242 medical services, from primary doctor visits to coronary angioplasty to foot x-ray."

So, what are you to do? Healthcare prices are crazy! Fortunately, the world is changing. There are a growing number of transparency tools for every healthcare industry sector (doctors, hospitals, and drugs) that you can access. This will help you pull the curtain back on the Great Wizard of Oz of healthcare.

---

23 Kodjak, Alison. "That Surgery Might Cost You A Lot Less In Another Town." NPR. April 27, 2016. Accessed April 19, 2018. https://www.npr.org/sections/health-shots/2016/04/27/475880565/that-surgery-might-cost-you-a-lot-less-in-another-town.

There are categories of transparency sites. The first is what I call qualitative sites. They provide useful information such as: areas of specialty, college education, hospital affiliation, ease of scheduling, staff responsiveness, patient level of trust, and amount of time spent with patient. These sites are useful in helping determine the type of relationship you might have with your doctor.

VISIT THESE SITES TO FIND QUALITATIVE INFORMATION RELATING TO DOCTORS

For doctors, some of the more popular websites include the following:

- WebMD.com
- Yelp.com
- Healthgrades.com
- RateMDs.com
- Vitals.com
- CareDash.com

The second set of sites focus more on the quantitative, or outcome-based, aspects of the doctor's care. For example, they examine items such as costs and how the doctor ranks against his/her peer set for a procedure. Does the doctor you're reviewing perform more or fewer procedures than their peers? This is important. Remember Malcolm Gladwell's position that the more you practice the better you are. The following websites provide you access to healthcare transparency.

---

24   Guroo is an affiliate of HCCI (Healthcare Cost Institute).

- GoodRX.com
- OneRX.com
- SingleCare.com
- RXhope.com

Note: I haven't found one single resource that has provided every answer or covered every area of the country yet, but these resources are growing, becoming more robust, and currently providing us more access to the real costs than we have ever had before. USE them. When comparing costs, look outside your area and see if your situation turns out like the knee replacement from Sacramento to Tucson or if your hospital has substandard records on the services you need covered.

If you're on your employer's health plan, ask to see if the health insurance carrier provides a price calculator and quality evaluation tool. If not, ask your employer to investigate offering one. Companies like Castlight, Amino Health, or Grand Rounds can be added, offering access to transparency. Remember, if you save yourself money, you save your employer money, too. They will direct you to the most cost-effective provider based on that carrier's network and negotiated discounts.

"Nobody spends somebody else's money as carefully as he spends his own. Nobody uses somebody else's resources as carefully as he uses his own. So if you want efficiency and effectiveness, if you want knowledge to be properly utilized, you have to do it through the means of private property."

—Milton Friedman (1912–2006), American economist and statistician

When it comes to transparency, the genie is out of the bottle. If we seek it, demand it, and use it, there's no way they (the industry) can put it back in. Let's move on to some examples of how to do just that.

MILLENNIALS: THE FUTURE

The paradigm shifts with the millennials. Due to their age, they have not utilized the healthcare system. They are less inclined, like their parents and grandparents, to have preconceived notions of what it should deliver. They, like the baby boomer generation, are transformative. Their immersion in technology produces a proficiency and dependence on its use. They are used to using all the how-to tools to learn what they need to know. They will adopt and leverage healthcare transparency, and with that adoption, the healthcare system will change.

That's not to say that the rest of us will sit on the side-lines or can afford to sit on the sidelines. We just have more habits to break. Health costs and healthcare insurance premiums are becoming a significant portion of our household budgets. It's time for all of us to become discriminating consumers and seek out quality health-care at the best cost.

You have now completed the first and most important step in becoming an effective healthcare consumer and gaining control. You have profiled your health and potential expenses, determined how you're going to fund those expenses, and developed a checklist to assist in analyzing the various programs presented to you. You are now prepared to wade through the labyrinth of industry terms and jargon (second only to the US government).

WHOM DO YOU TRUST?

One obstacle to taking control of your health is wading through the alphabet soup created by the health insurance industry. Whether purposely or not, the industry has created its own complicated language. The industry uses more acronyms than the US government! Why so many? PPOs? HMOs? POSs? EPOs? HOAs? HSAs? It's obnoxious.

Whether you're looking on an insurance company website

or you're talking to someone about a plan, they'll inevitably start rattling off these acronyms. You'll wonder, "Whoa, wait a minute here. What the heck is going on? Was I supposed to learn another language?" They even try to make things simpler by categorizing plans as gold, silver, and bronze. Maybe it works, but once they throw in "PPOs" and say they're "HSA-compatible," it becomes overwhelming.

It's hard to tell if all the acronyms are intentionally confusing or not. It's complex and layered. ACA worked on simplifying it, but it has a long way to go.

There's also an emotional aspect to the choices provided by insurance companies that many people don't consider. For example, you're only given a window of thirty days to sign up during open enrollment—and sometimes even less. Open enrollment used to run from November to the end of February. Now, it's been shrunk to just the end of the year. That means you have a finite period of time to become an expert in something you likely don't have any interest in learning more about, so you end up rushing to make a choice on coverage. If you're already denying the reality that you might get sick, now you add in a short deadline, confusing terminology, and a great financial risk? It's enough to tick you off. Then, if you want to change coverage, you have to go to your previous provider to find your records. What if you can't find your password? You're already on a time crunch. The list of hang-ups goes on and on.

So, what do you do? Inevitably, most people just take whatever coverage they had last year because they don't want to think about it. The world didn't come to an end, they still had enough money to survive, and they're running out of time. It's a perfect equation for inertia against change. This is where you pull out your work on your health profile and have a clear idea of who you are health-wise, what your expenses might be, and how much you can afford to cover. But you don't have to go it alone.

If you're employed and offered employer benefit plan option(s), utilize the resources available: your employer-supplied enrollment guide, your HR representative, the carrier information, the online enrolment tool that may have calculators built in for plan design, and your analysis of some of the tools we have mentioned throughout this chapter.

If you are buying health insurance on your own, you can use healthcare.gov or websites like healthsherpa.com, or you can engage an insurance professional.

If you choose to engage with an insurance professional, there are a few factors you want to look at first. You want somebody who has a large volume of health business, is connected to all available markets so they can show you a comprehensive representation of the marketplace, and who can explore some of the alternative ideas we just discussed with you. You want someone who will talk one-on-one with you and explain your options. You want someone who will be available throughout the year for questions, clarification, or direction to the correct sources to assist. Many, if not most, of the agents are represented through online services. The right one can be of great value to you.

Now what? Speaking of insurance, let's move on to part 2 of this book. What is covered, what does it cost, and how do you get it? Stay with me.

PART II

WHAT IS COVERED? WHAT DOES IT COST? WHERE DO I GET IT? UNDERSTANDING YOUR INSURANCE OPTIONS

CHAPTER SEVEN

WHY IS INSURANCE IMPORTANT?

You have completed a Health Risk Assessment identifying what health issues you have or may have because of family history. You have taken a look at what current costs are for those conditions. You have been exposed to catastrophic costs. You have sized up your financial situation. You have determined transferring that risk is worth consideration. You have walked through the seven steps on how to quantify your health insurance costs. You now have a basic understanding of your needs and how to analyze costs. It's time to dig deeper under the hood of healthcare insurance.

In part 2, we will explore:

- Coverage types (essentially covered benefits, plan types)
- Premium costs (direct, employer-sponsored, and government subsidies)
- Tax incentives (direct or through an employer)
- Rules of the road (eligibility for coverage)

Each above section will be addressed from three approaches: if you are offered employer health insurance, if you are buying individually, or if you are buying through the government programs. We'll then cover supplemental and nontraditional alternatives.

WARNING

The material in this section is why insurance gets a bad name. It is technical and dry, full of industry jargon and acronyms foreign to almost all. But it's what you'll be presented with when selecting health insurance and what you need to know. Hopefully, the format will provide that GPS directional assistance clarifying the clutter. Good Luck.

WHAT DO INSURANCE PLANS COVER?

The Affordable Care Act (ACA), aka Obamacare, mandated all individual or employer-sponsored health plans must cover these ten essential benefits without annual or lifetime spending caps. Note: annual deductibles, copays, and out-of-pocket requirements must still be met, but once met, the medical expense cannot be limited.

- Ambulatory patient services (outpatient care without being admitted to the hospital)
- Emergency services
- Hospitalization (such as surgery and overnight stays)
- Pregnancy, maternity, and newborn care (both before and after birth)
- Mental health and substance abuse disorder services including behavioral health treatment
- Prescription drugs
- Rehabilitation and habilitative services (those that help patients acquire, maintain, or improve skills necessary for daily functioning) and devices
- Laboratory services
- Preventive and wellness services and chronic disease management
- Pediatric services, including oral and vision

In addition, a set of preventive services for men, women, and children are covered at 100 percent under the plans without charging copays, deductibles, or out-of-pocket costs. These include annual physicals, female contraceptives, and immunizations. For a list of all 100 percent covered services go to healthcare.gov. If you have coverage through your employer, ask for and review your employer's Summary Plan Description (SPD).

Remember: The most efficient way to determine if your item is covered is to ask for the health insurance policy's "not covered" or "exclusion" section.

MINIMUM COVERAGE

Plans must cover the ten essential required benefits at an actuarial value of no less than 60 percent. Plans offered through healthcare.gov simplified the selection process by branding all plans that comply with the minimum 60 percent actuarial value as bronze plans.

noun: actuary; plural noun: actuaries

a person who compiles and analyzes statistics and uses them to calculate insurance risks and premiums.[25]

This is not to say that all healthcare insurance plans only cover the 60/40 percent split. There are 90/10 (platinum), 80/20 (gold), 70/30 (silver), and even some 50/50 (bronze as well) plans that comply with minimum actuarial value. Deductibles, copays, and maximum out-of-pocket expenses will vary by plan offering.

---

25   Google Dictionary's definition

Note: What are medically necessary charges? Medicare's definition of medically necessary charges is "health-related services or supplies needed to prevent, diagnose, or treat an illness, injury, condition, disease or its symptoms, and that meet accepted standards of medicine." In general terms, it excludes experimental unapproved procedures, and cosmetic procedures.[26]

WHAT PHYSICIANS AND HOSPITALS (MEDICAL PROVIDERS) ARE COVERED?

So far, we have highlighted what procedures are covered. You must also consider which providers are covered. Whatever plan or plans you are presented with and are considering, make sure they offer the doctors or hospitals or facilities that you are using. Different types of plans (HMO, PPO) and different insurance carriers (Blue Cross Blue Shield, Aetna, Cigna, United Healthcare, etc.) represent different providers. Some plans have more doctors and hospitals available and others fewer. Some may be limited by geographic areas.

How do you find out if your providers are available? Ask for the provider directory. Each insurance carrier's plan has its own unique list or directory. All are available online. You are given the option to review

---

26 Medicare.gov. (2018). *Medicare.gov: the official U.S. government site for Medicare | Medicare.* [online] Available at: https://www.medicare.gov/ [Accessed 24 Oct. 2018].

the provider directories when you are applying for the insurance. Health insurance carriers, employer plans, and government-sponsored plans offer multiple types of plans each with their own unique provider directory. When looking for your provider(s) in the carrier's directory, make sure you are looking at the correct health plan. Different plans within the same carrier will have different lists of providers.

TIP

If you don't have a doctor relationship established, you need to ask how many doctors in the plan you are choosing are accepting new patients. Doctors on the list may not be taking new patients. Ask the insurance company or pick a doctor and call them to ask if they are taking new patients under the plan you are looking to select.

CHAPTER EIGHT

WHAT ARE YOUR OPTIONS?

Roughly 289 million people in America have some kind of health plan. That leaves about 9 percent of the population not covered, meaning we have a 91 percent coverage rate. We get our health insurance from the following sources: we enroll in our employer-offered plans, we directly purchase from insurance carriers ourselves, we qualify for and enroll in Medicaid, we turn sixty-five and enroll in Medicare, or we are employed through a government entity and receive one of their offerings. Obamacare (ACA) has been successful in increasing the number of Americans with health insurance by subsidizing the cost through income-based subsidies for insurance and increasing participation in Medicaid. It has standardized the types of plans offered and removed previous barriers to purchasing insurance, like preexisting conditions. What it has not done is simplify or reduce the cost.[27] We are going to address:

1. What types of plans are available and which source offers them?
2. Who pays for the monthly premiums and how much?
3. Are there tax-incentivized plans and how do I take advantage of them?
4. When, where, and how do I enroll?

PLAN TYPES

The current marketplace offers choices among these four basic plan structures: Preferred Provider Organization (PPO), Health Maintenance Organization (HMO), and High-Deductible Health Plans (HDHP), which can be coupled with a Health Savings Account (HSA) and Health Reimbursement Account plans. It's important to understand the basic features and differences among plan types. Whatever source you have been provided to review benefits should clearly identify itself as one of these plan types. The plan types address what the plans cover (like what hospitals and doctors are available, whether doctor visits require referrals, and any tax savings opportuni-

---

27 "Health Insurance Coverage of the Total Population." The Henry J. Kaiser Family Foundation. September 19, 2017. Accessed April 17, 2018. https://www.kff.org/other/state-indicator/total-population/.

ties) versus what you have to pay to participate in the plan (deductibles, copays, and out-of-pocket costs).

Let's review the basic health insurance plan features incorporated in the plan types.

PROVIDER NETWORKS

A provider network is a list of doctors and other health-care providers and hospitals that a health insurer has contracted with to provide medical care to its members at discounted rates. These providers are called "network providers" or "in-network providers." Why would providers offer a discount for their services? Because the insurers pass some of the provider discounts to its members to reduce the cost of the members' monthly premiums and out-of-pocket costs for in-network services. Note that in the examples provided for each plan type, the in-network deductibles and out-of-pocket limits are half of the out-of-network costs.

REFRESHER COURSE

Copay: Your copay is a predetermined rate you pay for specifically listed healthcare services at the time of care. You won't have any other payment. For example, you may have a $25 copay every time you see your primary care physician. All you pay is $25 even though the doctor may bill your plan more than this.

Deductible: The deductible is how much you pay before your health insurance starts to cover a larger portion of your bills. Deductibles usually come in individual and family categories. If you have an individual (single) plan, you must meet the individual deductible before the plan begins to pay for the cost of services. If you have a family plan, the plan will begin to pay on any one individual as soon as that individual reaches the individual deductible. When medical claims from all family members exceed the family deductible level, any other claim from any two family members will be eligible for the plan to pay. The deductible resets yearly.

Coinsurance: Coinsurance is a percentage of a medical charge that you pay, with the rest paid by your health insurance plan, after your deductible has been met. For example, if you have an 80/20 percent coinsurance plan, your health insurance will cover 80 percent and you will pay 20 percent of each covered medical bill after meeting the deductible. Common coinsurance arrangements are 90/10, 80/20, 70/30, and 60/40.

Out-of-pocket maximum: The most you could have to pay in one year, out of pocket, for your healthcare before your insurance covers 100 percent of the bill. The maximum out-of-pocket for any accredited ACA plan is $7,900 for an individual plan and $15,800 for a family plan (2019). The same principles governing the family deductible apply to the family out-of-pocket maximum.

Important: Deductible, coinsurance, and out-of-pocket maximum categories express coverage offerings by individual or family coverage. The difference is somewhat self-explanatory—the individual is for one person; the family is for two or more. Most think the entire family deductible must be met before the plan begins to pay, but this is not accurate. Each individual only pays a deductible up to the individual deductible level; each family as a group only pays up to the family deductible level.

Each plan type (PPO, HMO, HDHP, and HRA) could have multiple levels of out-of-pocket costs to you. For example, you might be presented with two PPO plans, one with a $2,000 individual deductible and $4,000 individual maximum out-of-pocket costs, and one with $4,000 individual deductible and $8,000 individual maximum out-of-pocket costs. Both plans are PPOs. The plans commonly apply names like Platinum, Gold, Silver, and Bronze to highlight the differences in your out-of-pocket costs. The seven-step cost spend analysis prepared you to determine the appropriate financial risk you can manage. Let's now explore what plan types make sense for you.

PREFERRED PROVIDER PLANS (PPO)

PPOs are available in most geographic areas of the country in all three approaches: employer-sponsored plans, direct individual plans, and government plans. The name of the plan type "preferred provider" tells you about the key characteristic of the plan. PPOs grant you the freedom of choice to see any provider but create a network of physicians and hospitals ("in-network") that offer discounted pricing to plan members. The networks are generally broad but do not include all providers. The sample PPO plan shows two columns of benefits: In-Network Benefits and Out-of-Network Benefits. Note the doubling of the out-of-network deductibles and maximum out-of-pocket costs. This is to incentivize you to use the providers who are offering the network a discount. PPOs generally offer both deductibles and copays—charges you are required to pay. The PPO premiums tend to be higher than HMO plans.

PPO Plan Benefit Summary

GENERAL PLAN INFORMATION	IN-NETWORK BENEFITS	OUT-OF-NETWORK BENEFITS
Annual Deductible/Individual	$1,000	$2,000
Annual Deductible/Family	$2,000	$4,000
Coinsurance (Who Pays)	80% Plan; 20% You	60% Plan; 40% You
Office Visit/Exam	$30 copay	You pay 40% after deductible
Outpatient Specialist Visit	$50 copay	You pay 40% after deductible
Annual Out-of-Pocket Limit/Individual	$5,000	$10,000
Annual Out-of-Pocket Limit/Family	$10,000	$20,000
Lifetime Plan Maximum	Unlimited	Unlimited

INPATIENT HOSPITAL SERVICES

	IN-NETWORK	OUT-OF-NETWORK
Inpatient Hospitalization	You pay 20% after deductible	You pay 40% after deductible
Semi-Private Room & Board	You pay 20% after deductible	You pay 40% after deductible
(Including services and supplies)		

EMERGENCY SERVICES

	IN-NETWORK	OUT-OF-NETWORK
Emergency Room	$250 Copay, waived if admitted	$250 Copay, waived if admitted

MENTAL HEALTH BENEFITS

	IN-NETWORK	OUT-OF-NETWORK
Inpatient Care	You pay 20% after deductible	You pay 40% after deductible
Outpatient Care	$30 Copay	You pay 40% after deductible

ALCOHOL ABUSE

Inpatient Care

	IN-NETWORK	OUT-OF-NETWORK
Inpatient Hospitalization	You pay 20% after deductible	You pay 40% after deductible

Outpatient Care

	IN-NETWORK	OUT-OF-NETWORK
Outpatient Services	$30 copay	You pay 40% after deductible

GENERAL PLAN INFORMATION	IN-NETWORK BENEFITS	OUT-OF-NETWORK BENEFITS
SUBSTANCE ABUSE		
Inpatient Care		
Inpatient Hospitalization	You pay 20% after deductible	You pay 40% after deductible
Outpatient Care	$30 copay	You pay 40% after deductible
Outpatient Services		
PRESCRIPTION DRUG BENEFITS		
Prescription Drug Deductible	N/A	N/A
Generic	$10 copay	Not covered
Brand (Formulary/Preferred)	$30 copay	Not covered
Brand (Non-Formulary/Non-Preferred)	$50 copay	Not covered
Number of Days' Supply	31 days	31 days
Mail Order		
Mail Order	Not mandatory	Not mandatory
Generic	$20 copay	Not covered
Brand (Formulary/Preferred)	$60 copay	Not covered
Brand (Non-Formulary/Non-Preferred)	$100 copay	Not covered
Number of Days' Supply for Mail Order	90 days	N/A
Other Services and Supplies		You pay 40% after deductible
Chiropractic Services	$30 copay, 20 visits per year	Max 20 visits per year

The above information is intended as a benefit summary only. It does not include all of the benefit provisions, limitations, and qualifications. If this information conflicts in any way with the contract, the contract will prevail.

Caution: Be aware of "balanced billing" if you go to out-of-network providers. Balanced billing means you will be responsible for any charges above what the insurance company will cover, even if you have met your maximum out-of-pocket costs. If you are considering using an out-of-network provider, check with your plan on how it pays those providers.

HEALTH MAINTENANCE ORGANIZATION (HMO)

HMOs are available in all three approaches: employer-sponsored plans, direct individual plans, and government plans. Their goal, by managing the care and access to care, is to deliver better benefits at a lower premium than other plans.

Access to Care

HMOs offer a contracted network of physicians and medical providers that you may choose. There is no coverage for non-networked providers (except in emergencies). They limit their networks to select providers in exchange for deeper discounts on those providers' services. This allows them to pass along reduced costs to you.

Note the following: HMO networks can be limited to certain geographic areas. If you travel or have family members living in different locations (e.g., college students), make sure the HMO network has providers where you are traveling. In addition, their networks are smaller. Make sure the doctors you are using now and the type of doctors you might need (refer to your health profile) are available in their network.

Managed Care

Some HMOs manage your care by requiring you to select a primary care physician (PCP) who determines what treatment you need. Referrals from the PCP to other medical service providers within the network may be required in order for the plan to pay benefits.

Benefits

As you can see in the HMO example, your out-of-pocket expenses are expressed in a copay for services versus deductibles. This allows you to know exactly what you will spend for each service, making it much easier to budget. Once your copays exceed the annual spending limit, the plan pays claims at 100 percent. Copay amounts will differ by plan. The higher the copay amounts, the lower the monthly premium.

In a nutshell, in exchange for having HMOs manage your care with a selective network of healthcare providers, you are offered lower monthly premiums with lower out-of-pocket costs. Certainly, this idea is one worth investigating.

HMO Benefit Summary

GENERAL PLAN INFORMATION	NETWORK BENEFITS
Annual Deductible/Individual	$0
Annual Deductible/Family	$0
Coinsurance (Who Pays)	100% Plan, after OOP Limit
Office Visit/Exam	$10 copay
Outpatient Specialist Visit	$10 copay
Annual Out-of-Pocket Limit/Individual	$1,500
Annual Out-of-Pocket Limit/Family	$3,000
Lifetime Plan Maximum	Unlimited

INPATIENT HOSPITAL SERVICES

Inpatient Hospitalization	100%
Semi-Private Room & Board	100%

(Including services and supplies)

EMERGENCY SERVICES

Emergency Room	$50 copay, waived if admitted

MENTAL HEALTH BENEFITS

Inpatient Care	100%
Outpatient Care	$10 copay

ALCOHOL ABUSE

Inpatient Care

Inpatient Hospitalization	100%

GENERAL PLAN INFORMATION	NETWORK BENEFITS

Outpatient Care

Outpatient Services	$10 copay

SUBSTANCE ABUSE

Inpatient Care

Inpatient Hospitalization	100%

Outpatient Care

Outpatient Services	$10 copay

PRESCRIPTION DRUG BENEFITS

Prescription Drug Deductible	N/A
Generic	$10 copay
Brand (Formulary/Preferred)	$30 copay
Brand (Non-Formulary/Non-Preferred)	N/A
Number of Days' Supply	30 days

Mail Order

Mail Order	Not mandatory
Generic	$20 copay
Brand (Formulary/Preferred)	$60 copay
Brand (Non-Formulary/Non-Preferred)	N/A
Number of Days' Supply for Mail Order	100 days

OTHER SERVICES AND SUPPLIES

Chiropractic Services	Not covered

The above information is intended as a benefit summary only. It does not include all of the benefit provisions, limitations, and qualifications. If this information conflicts in any way with the contract, the contract will prevail.

HIGH-DEDUCTIBLE HEALTH PLANS WITH A HEALTH REIMBURSEMENT ACCOUNT (HRA)

Don't confuse this HRA with a Health Risk Assessment! Remember, health reimbursement accounts are only offered through employer health plans.

A Health Reimbursement Account's (HRA) features are attached to a PPO plan. They are an IRS-approved, employer-funded account for you to pay out-of-pocket health expenses. Its most common use is when employers introduce a higher deductible health plan and establish an HRA account for employees who select it. The account is used to offset out-of-pocket expenses (deductibles and coinsurance), thus reducing the financial burden on the employee. The employer has the sole discretion on how much it contributes, up to the maximum amount allowable. The deposited funds are generally available only for the plan year and, if not used, may not be rolled over to the following year. At the employer's discretion, funds can be rolled over and accumulated if not used.

Your employer's open enrollment material will clearly identify such a plan and its provisions in the material. If offered, it could be a viable way to entertain a higher deductible and coinsurance plan, which should reduce your monthly premium while softening the impact of a high deductible if claims materialize. You must remember that the money in the account is the employer's money and not yours. You cannot take it with you in the event you leave that employer. The funds revert back to the employer. So, HRAs are a good way to transition to a higher deductible plan and lower monthly premium costs, but they're not a long-term healthcare personal savings vehicle.

The next example highlights an HRA. As you can see, it looks just like the earlier PPO example, except for the employer HRA contribution of $1,000/individual and $2,000/family. This is the fund the employer sets up for you to use to offset your out-of-pocket costs. In essence, it reduces the $2,000 individual deductible to $1,000, and the family deductible from $4,000 to $2,000.

HRA Benefit Summary

GENERAL PLAN INFORMATION	IN-NETWORK BENEFITS	OUT-OF-NETWORK BENEFITS
Annual Deductible/Individual	$2,000	$4,000
Annual Deductible/Family	$4,000	$8,000
Coinsurance (Who Pays)	80% Plan; 20% You	60% Plan; 40% You
Office Visit/Exam	You pay 20% after deductible	You pay 40% after deductible
Outpatient Specialist Visit	You pay 20% after deductible	You pay 40% after deductible
Annual Out-of-Pocket Limit/Individual	$4,000	$8,000
Annual Out-of-Pocket Limit/Family	$8,000	$16,000
Lifetime Plan Maximum	Unlimited	Unlimited

EMPLOYER HRA CONTRIBUTION $1,000 INDIVIDUAL; $2,000 FAMILY

INPATIENT HOSPITAL SERVICES

Inpatient Hospitalization	You pay 20% after deductible	You pay 40% after deductible
Semi-Private Room & Board	You pay 20% after deductible	You pay 40% after deductible
(Including Services and Supplies)		

EMERGENCY SERVICES

Emergency Room	You pay 20% after deductible	You pay 40% after deductible

MENTAL HEALTH BENEFITS

Inpatient Care	You pay 20% after deductible	You pay 40% after deductible
Outpatient Care	You pay 20% after deductible	You pay 40% after deductible

ALCOHOL ABUSE

Inpatient Care

Inpatient Hospitalization	You pay 20% after deductible	You pay 40% after deductible

Outpatient Care

Outpatient Services	You pay 20% after deductible	You pay 40% after deductible

GENERAL PLAN INFORMATION	IN-NETWORK BENEFITS	OUT-OF-NETWORK BENEFITS

SUBSTANCE ABUSE

Inpatient Care

Inpatient Hospitalization	You pay 20% after deductible	You pay 40% after deductible

Outpatient Care

Outpatient Services	You pay 20% after deductible	You pay 40% after deductible

PRESCRIPTION DRUG BENEFITS

Prescription Drug Deductible	N/A	N/A
Generic	$10 copay	Not covered
Brand (Formulary/Preferred)	$30 copay	Not covered
Brand (Non-Formulary/ Non-Preferred)	$50 copay	Not covered
Number of Days' Supply	31 days	

Mail Order

Mail Order	Not mandatory	Not mandatory
Generic	$20 copay	Not covered
Brand (Formulary/Preferred)	$60 copay	Not covered
Brand (Non-Formulary/ Non-Preferred)	$100 copay	Not covered
Number of Days' Supply for Mail Order	90 days	

OTHER SERVICES AND SUPPLIES

Chiropractic Services	You pay 20% after deductible	You pay 40% after deductible
		Max 20 visits per year

The above information is intended as a benefit summary only. It does not include all of the benefit provisions, limitations, and qualifications. If this information conflicts in any way with the contract, the contract will prevail.

HIGH-DEDUCTIBLE HEALTH PLANS (HDHP) QUALIFIED FOR HEALTH SAVING ACCOUNTS (HSAs)

High-Deductible Health Plans that qualify for a Health Savings Account are available through employer-based plans and the direct insurance market. Currently, government programs do not offer HDHP plans with HSAs. The programs are becoming more prevalent with 70 percent of large employers offering at least one HDHP exclusively or as an option in 2018.[28]

A High-Deductible Health Plan follows all the features of a basic PPO with one exception: it cannot offer any copays for any level of service. The plans do not pay until deductibles are met; that includes physician office visits and prescription drugs (see example plan). Deductibles must be at least $1,350 for an individual and $2,700 for a family. They do, though, cover basic annual physicals at 100%.

Why would you consider such a plan? The first benefit is lower monthly premiums. The second is the opportunity to open a health savings account and save money on a before-tax basis. Qualified HDHPs are the only plans allowed to utilize health savings accounts. Unlike the HRA, the money you save is yours. It's like a 401(k) retirement plan. The amounts can grow, be invested, and stay with you when you leave your employer or retire. The funds can be used for healthcare expenses and health insurance premiums.

---

28 Miller, Stephen. "High-Deductible Plans More Common, but So Are Choices." SHRM. August 17, 2018. Accessed September 07, 2018. https://www.shrm.org/resourcesandtools/hr-topics/benefits/pages/high-deductible-plans-more-common-but-so-are-choices.aspx.

HDHP Benefit Summary

GENERAL PLAN INFORMATION	IN-NETWORK BENEFITS	OUT-OF-NETWORK BENEFITS
Annual Deductible/Individual	$1,350	$2,700
Annual Deductible/Family	$2,700	$5,400
Coinsurance (Who Pays)	80% Plan; 20% You	60% Plan; 40% You
Office Visit/Exam	You pay 20% after deductible	You pay 40% after deductible
Outpatient Specialist Visit	You pay 20% after deductible	You pay 40% after deductible
Annual Out-of-Pocket Limit/Individual	$4,000	$8,000
Annual Out-of-Pocket Limit/Family	$8,000	$16,000
Lifetime Plan Maximum	Unlimited	Unlimited

INPATIENT HOSPITAL SERVICES

Inpatient Hospitalization	You pay 20% after deductible	You pay 40% after deductible
Semi-Private Room & Board	You pay 20% after deductible	You pay 40% after deductible
(Including services and supplies)		

EMERGENCY SERVICES

Emergency Room	You pay 20% after deductible	You pay 40% after deductible

MENTAL HEALTH BENEFITS

Inpatient Care	You pay 20% after deductible	You pay 40% after deductible
Outpatient Care	You pay 20% after deductible	You pay 40% after deductible

ALCOHOL ABUSE

Inpatient Care

Inpatient Hospitalization	You pay 20% after deductible	You pay 40% after deductible

Outpatient Care

Outpatient Services	You pay 20% after deductible	You pay 40% after deductible

GENERAL PLAN INFORMATION	IN-NETWORK BENEFITS	OUT-OF-NETWORK BENEFITS

SUBSTANCE ABUSE

Inpatient Care

Inpatient Hospitalization	You pay 20% after deductible	You pay 40% after deductible

Outpatient Care

Outpatient Services	You pay 20% after deductible	You pay 40% after deductible

PRESCRIPTION DRUG BENEFITS

Prescription Drug Deductible	$0	$0
Generic	You pay 20% after deductible	Not covered
Brand (Formulary/Preferred)	You pay 20% after deductible	Not covered
Brand (Non-Formulary/Non-Preferred)	You pay 20% after deductible	Not covered
Number of Days' Supply	31 days	

Mail Order

Mail Order Mandatory	Not mandatory	Not mandatory
Generic	You pay 20% after deductible	Not covered
Brand (Formulary/Preferred)	You pay 20% after deductible	Not covered
Brand (Non-Formulary/Non-Preferred)	You pay 20% after deductible	Not covered
Number of Days' Supply for Mail Order	90 days	

OTHER SERVICES AND SUPPLIES

Chiropractic Services	You pay 20% after deductible	You pay 40% after deductible
		Max 20 visits per year

The above information is intended as a benefit summary only. It does not include all of the benefit provisions, limitations, and qualifications. If this information conflicts in any way with the contract, the contract will prevail.

CASE STUDY

Tracy, the poster child for knowing how to manage your risk, was constantly battling health issues; she had horrible, debilitating rheumatoid arthritis and had undergone surgery on her feet. She constantly had to take many specialty medications. She had guaranteed ongoing medical expenses—and lots of them. Health insurance was a major necessity for her.

Back in about 2005—before the ACA, remember—Tracy was offered two PPO plans and her employer introduced a $5,000 individual maximum out-of-pocket HDHP with an HSA account. The plan was structured such that once employees reached the $5,000 deductible, the plan paid 100 percent of all expenses. This was $1,000 less than the PPO plan, but it didn't offer drug copays or doctor visit copays. For the first two years, Tracy's employer contributed $1,000 to an employee HSA account, and the monthly premiums of the HDHP were 20 percent less than the PPO plan.

Tracy did the math. She figured out that the combined costs of her monthly prescription and doctor office visits would exceed her total deductible and out-of-pocket requirements under the HDHP by mid-year. She would, at that point, receive 100 percent benefits. Couple that with the 20 percent reduction in premium cost that she could apply to her HSA, and the $1,000 employer contribution, and she would end up *saving* money.

The downside to Tracy's plan was that, yes, she'd have to front the money—which, quite frankly, was tight at best, like it is for most of us. Not wanting to give up the savings due to a cash flow shortfall, she got creative and went to her doctors. She asked for payment plans, which they all accepted. She even negotiated some reductions in costs.

Tracy became a proactive consumer of her healthcare!

PRESCRIPTION DRUG COVERAGE

All ACA-approved plans must cover prescription drugs. Different plans cover them at different levels, but there are universal prescription drug features you should be familiar with.

A drug formulary is a list of drugs covered by your health plan. They include Food and Drug Administration-approved generic, brand-name, and specialty drugs. Plans generally offer different levels of copays for the different drug categories. Generally, generic drugs have the lowest copays and specialty drugs have the highest. Some plans will not cover drugs that are non-formulary. Others cover them, but you are required to pay a higher copay.

CHAPTER NINE

WHO PAYS FOR WHAT?

You do. But that does not mean necessarily that you are paying 100 percent of the cost. There are three basic categories of health insurance sources: employers, individuals buying health insurance, and government programs. Employer-sponsored plans represent groups of people which translate to volume for the insurance carriers. Volume allows for greatest flexibility with plan designs, access to broader provider networks (hospitals and physicians), and pricing.

COVERAGE THROUGH YOUR EMPLOYER

Employer coverage is pretty straightforward: you work for somebody, they offer coverage, they pay for a majority of the premium, and you enroll. Employers with over fifty employees are required by the ACA to offer healthcare coverage to their full-time employees (those working over thirty hours per week) or pay a $2,000 penalty for each full-time employee every year. Most elect to offer the coverage. They must offer at least one plan that complies with all ACA guidelines, including the essential coverage, the minimum plan design, and maximum employee monthly contribution of 9.86 percent of household monthly income for 2019 single coverage. Employers with fewer than fifty employees have the option to offer coverage or not; it depends on their financial situation. If you work for an employer who does not offer coverage, you will need to investigate options: purchasing directly or, depending on your financial situation, looking into government-sponsored plans.

TIP

ACA allows children to stay on their parent's healthcare plan until age twenty-six. This is probably their best option.

PLAN OPTIONS

Most employers offer multiple options for their employees. The range of options addresses plan designs that impact how much is covered and what you'll have to spend if and when you use the healthcare system. Your premium contributions impact how much of your paycheck is paid monthly for your selected coverage. The options you are presented will be from the coverages we discussed (PPO, HMO, HDHP/ HSA). Many offer tax-deferred savings vehicles to help offset the cost of healthcare.

INDIVIDUALS BUYING DIRECTLY

Buying health insurance directly under Obamacare has been like trading one nightmare for another. Before Obamacare, people with existing conditions were denied coverage. With Obamacare, those people can now buy coverage, but more and more often they can't pay for the insurance coverage or find coverage. Many of the national health carriers (Anthem, Cigna, Aetna, United Healthcare) have reduced the number of states to which they offer individual health insurance to the point that a number of counties had only one health insurance carrier option in 2019. And increasingly, the options offered have smaller provider (hospital and physician) networks. Bottom line: if you are buying directly, you will probably need to consider increasing your deductibles and out-of-pocket costs to offset premium increases.

The Kaiser Family Foundation, www.kff.org, does an excellent job of tracking health insurance carriers offering coverage by state and the premium rate increases or decreases filed by health plans in each state. They are already compiling 2019 health insurance carrier

Doesn't Obamacare provide premium subsidies for non-government health insurance to offset the cost? Yes, it does. Obamacare provides premium tax credits and cost sharing subsidies. A portion of the monthly health premiums may be offset for individuals earning less than 400 percent of the federal poverty level (FPL). Interestingly, 84 percent of the people who signed up for individual health insurance since 2014 received subsidies. Luckily, because of inflation protection in the ACA subsidies, inflation increases (like 2018's 33–38 percent) are not passed on to those with subsidies. Their subsidies increased as the premium increased, keeping them whole. The people who bore the brunt of the increases were those without subsidies, and not all of them are rich.

Once again, Kaiser Family Foundation is an excellent
source for details regarding premium tax credits and
cost-sharing subsidies.[30]

The most efficient way to find out what plans, pricing,

29 "Key Facts about the Uninsured Population." *The Henry J. Kaiser Family Foundation*, 7 Dec.
2017, www.kff.org/uninsured/fact-sheet/key-facts-about-the-uninsured-population/.

30 "Total Marketplace Enrollment and Financial Assistance." *The Henry J. Kaiser
Family Foundation*, 13 June 2017, www.kff.org/health-reform/state-indicator/
total-marketplace-enrollment-and-financial-assistance/.

and subsidies are available to you is to access Health-care.gov or your state-sponsored healthcare exchange. Healthcare.gov covers thirty-seven states and the District of Columbia, and will direct you to state-sponsored exchanges. They will start the session by asking basic financial questions that will determine whether you qualify for a subsidy. In 2019, persons earning up to $48,560 may qualify for an individual's health insurance subsidy while individuals earning up to $83,120 may qualify for a family health insurance subsidy. The dollar amounts are adjusted annually.[31]

States with their own exchanges are: California, Colorado, Connecticut, District of Columbia, Idaho, Maryland, Massachusetts, Minnesota, New Mexico, Rhode Island, Vermont, and Washington.

Healthcare.gov got off to a rocky start in 2014. It has made great improvements since then but could still stand improvements in customer service. An alternative is Healthsherpa.com,[32] which covers all states and all available health plans. They are a private company whose mission statement is "to help every American feel the comfort and security of having health coverage. [They]

31 "The Henry J. Kaiser Family Foundation." The Henry J. Kaiser Family Foundation. Accessed September 25, 2018. https://www.kff.org/.

32 "Hello, We Are HealthSherpa." HealthSherpa | About HealthSherpa. Accessed April 19, 2018. https://www.healthsherpa.com/about.

use design, technology, and customer service by real people to make insurance easier to understand, faster to sign up, and simpler to use." The major differences are an easier and faster system, and real-time help. They provide counselors via chat rooms who walk through your enrollment and continue the chat room assistance throughout the year. They also have phone lines for those of us that would still like to talk directly with a counselor. These are game changers, and the use of their service is growing every year. In 2018, they enrolled 1 million members, or 10 percent of all individual insureds. Inside information is that many of the insurance agents and brokers use Sherpa as their back-room service model. So, why not try them direct?

GOVERNMENT PROGRAMS

Note that the following information is true as I write this book, but—as we all know—nothing stays the same, especially in the government and in the world of healthcare. Visit www.healthcare.gov for the most up-to-date information about the status of the healthcare system in the US and what it means to you.

MEDICAID

Medicaid is a joint federal and state program that, together with the Children's Health Insurance Program, makes up the single largest source of health coverage in the United States. Its goal is to provide low-income individuals, families, and children health insurance with little or no premiums, and little or no out-of-pocket medical expenses.

The Affordable Care Act of 2010 created the opportunity for states to expand Medicaid to cover nearly all low-income Americans under age sixty-five. Eligibility for children was extended to at least 133 percent of the federal poverty level (FPL) in every state (most states cover children to higher income levels), and states were given the option to extend eligibility to adults with income at or below 133 percent of the FPL. The majority of states have chosen to expand coverage to adults, and those that have not yet expanded may choose to do so at any time. Eighteen states have not expanded coverage as of 2019. They are Alabama, Florida, Georgia, Idaho, Kansas, Mississippi, Missouri, Nebraska, North Carolina, Oklahoma, South Carolina, South Dakota, Tennessee, Texas, Utah, Virginia, Wisconsin, and Wyoming.[33]

The 2019 federal poverty level (FPL) income numbers[34]

33 "A 50-State Look at Medicaid Expansion." Families USA. June 05, 2018. Accessed September 25, 2018. https://familiesusa.org/product/50-state-look-medicaid-expansion.

34 "Poverty Guidelines." ASPE. February 12, 2019. Accessed March 04, 2019. https://aspe.hhs.gov/poverty-guidelines.

are used to calculate eligibility for Medicaid and the Children's Health Insurance Program (CHIP).

2019 Federal Poverty Levels

HOUSEHOLD SIZE	48 CONTIGUOUS UNITED STATES	ALASKA	HAWAII
Individuals	$12,490	$15,600	$14,380
Family of 2	$16,910	$21,130	$19,460
Family of 3	$21,330	$26,660	$24,540
Family of 4	$25,750	$32,190	$29,620
Family of 5	$30,170	$37,720	$34,700
Family of 6	$34,590	$43,250	$39,780
Family of 7	$39,010	$48,780	$44,860
Family of 8	$43,430	$54,310	$49,940

Medicaid Benefits

States establish and administer their own Medicaid programs and determine the type, amount, duration, and scope of services within broad federal guidelines. Federal law requires states to provide certain mandatory benefits and allows states the choice of covering other optional benefits. Mandatory benefits include services like inpatient and outpatient hospital services, physician services, laboratory and x-ray services, and home health services, among others. Optional benefits include services like prescription drugs, case management, physical therapy, and occupational therapy.

You can enroll through healthcare.gov. Additional state-by-state information is on medicaid.gov. Or, you can try the American Council on Aging's Medicaid Assistance site at medicaidplanningassistance.org/state-medicaid-resources. They provide state-by-state names and contact info, and free planning advisor services.

CHILDREN'S HEALTH INSURANCE PROGRAM (CHIP)

Children's Health Insurance Program (CHIP) is a federal/state health program managed by the states. It provides medical coverage for individuals under age nineteen whose parents earn too much income to qualify for Medicaid, but not enough to pay for private coverage. Program coverage varies from state to state, but all states' CHIP plans cover routine checkups, immunizations, doctor visits, prescriptions, dental care, vision care, hospital care, laboratory services, x-rays, and emergency services. Some states also cover parents and pregnant women. Its goal, like Medicaid, is to provide health insurance with inexpensive or no premiums or out-of-pocket medical expenses.

It's cumbersome to get coverage through CHIP, but it could be a huge winner for your family if you qualify. If you make up to $40,000 for, say, a family of three, you can still get Medicaid coverage. CHIP, on the other hand, is for people who make more than that but still have a tough time affording coverage. We run into plenty of people who keep their employer's coverage for themselves but carve off their kids and put them on CHIP. To sign up, you can call 1-800-318-2596, or you can begin the process by completing an insurance application on healthcare.gov. The application will determine if you qualify for the program and will notify your state agency. Your state agency will contact you about enrollment. My advice is to do both and follow up.

Additional information is available through medicaid.gov.

MEDICARE

Medicare is the guaranteed-issue, government health insurance program for individuals over sixty-five, certain younger people with disabilities, and people with End Stage Renal Disease (permanent kidney failure requiring dialysis or transplant). It does not have income requirements to join. Its goal is similar to Medicaid in providing affordable healthcare insurance to seniors. All four components of Medicare (Parts A, B, C, and D) require monthly premiums, deductibles, and out-of-pocket costs for services.

Different parts of Medicare help cover specific services:

- Part A: Hospital Insurance. It covers inpatient hospital

stays, some home healthcare, stays in skilled nursing facilities, and hospice care.

- Part B: Medical Insurance. It covers outpatient care, preventive services, medical supplies, and some doctors' services.
- Part C: Medicare Advantage Plans. These are offered by private companies that contract with Medicare. They provide Part A and Part B coverage, and most also cover Part D benefits.
- Part D: Prescription Drug Coverage. This is provided by private insurance companies and adds drug coverage to the other parts of Medicare.

Additional information is available at medicare.gov, or for supplemental assistance and supplemental policies, consult the American Association of Retired Persons (AARP).

TAKING ADVANTAGE OF TAX-SAVING INCENTIVES

Health insurance and healthcare expenses can cost a fortune. If the IRS offers tax-incentivized plans, you need to take advantage of them. If not, it's like throwing money away.

EMPLOYER-OFFERED TAX-SAVINGS PLANS

Your employer may elect to offer two additional tax-advantaged or pre-tax programs where you can deduct money from your paycheck before taxes, thus increasing your purchasing power and reducing your taxes. They are:

1. The premium-only plan (POP) that lets you pay for your monthly portion of the premiums pre-tax; and
2. The Flexible Spending Account (FSA) that allows you to save money from your paycheck on a pre-tax basis toward medical expenses for the year. You can consult tasconline.com, a company for employers providing flexible spending account administrative services, and search for eligible expenses for a complete list of eligible charges. Your employer will decide the amount you may save, up to a max of $2,650/year in 2018. Eligible expenses include your healthcare plan's copays, deductibles, and coinsurance. Medications are covered as long as they are prescribed by your doctor. The catch with FSAs is that you have to either use the funds in the plan year or lose them to your employer. That sounds unfair, right? Well, maybe not. The FSA rules allow you to access 100 percent of what you committed to save for the year at any time during the year, meaning you can access the full year before you have saved for it. Therefore, you need to accurately assess what your expenses will be to ensure you don't waste your money. There has been a slight loosening of the "lose it" provision, and at this time, you can carry $500 forward into future years.

There is no reason for you not to take the POP plan and reduce your cost of the monthly premium. You should be aware, though, that if you elect to take the POP, you cannot drop the health coverage until the next open enrollment unless you have a qualifying life event (QLE). The FSA, likewise, is an excellent way to reduce your costs if you know which medical expenses you will be incurring in the coming year. Why pay more for the services or more to the government in taxes?

EMPLOYER AND INDIVIDUAL TAX INCENTIVE PLANS—HEALTH SAVINGS ACCOUNT (HSA)

Health Savings Accounts are available in both the individual and employer markets if you have elected a High-Deductible Health Plan (HDHP; see plan types in this book). High-deductible health plans with HSAs do have minimum deductible and maximum out-of-pocket expense requirements for individual-only and family coverage. The 2019 levels are as follows: $1,350 for individual coverage and $2,700 for family coverage, in terms of the minimum annual deductible. The maximum annual deductible and other out-of-pocket expense limits are $6,750 for individual coverage and $13,500 for family coverage.

Benefits of an HSA

The following are benefits of an HSA:

- You can claim a tax deduction for contributions you, or someone other than your employer, make to your HSA even if you don't itemize your deductions on a Schedule A (Form 1040).
- Contributions to your HSA made by your employer (including contributions made through a cafeteria plan) may be excluded from your gross income.
- The contributions remain in your account until you use them.
- The interest or other earnings on the assets in the account are tax free.
- You can save tax free and distributions may be tax free if used to pay qualified medical expenses.
- An HSA is "portable." It stays with you if you change employers or leave the workforce.

HSA Contribution Limits

For individuals buying insurance directly, HSA regulations allow you to legally reduce federal income tax up to $3,500 a year for individuals, or $7,000 for families, into a health savings account for tax year 2019, as long as you're covered by an HSA-qualified HDHP. There's no minimum deposit, but whatever you put into your account is an "above the line" tax deduction that reduces your adjusted gross income. Just like IRAs, HSA contributions can be made until April 15 of the following year. Account holders who are fifty-five or older are allowed to deposit an additional $1,000 in catch-up contributions (this amount is not adjusted for inflation; it's always $1,000).

For people with employer-sponsored HDHP/HSA accounts, they can deduct up to the same amounts from their payroll before taxes are taken out.

Using Your HSA Funds

You can use the tax-free savings in your HSA to pay for doctor visits, hospital costs, deductibles, copays, prescription drugs, or any other qualified medical expenses. Once the out-of-pocket maximum on your health insurance policy is met, your health insurance plan will pay for your remaining covered medical expenses, the same as any other health plan.

If you switch to a health insurance policy that's not HSA-qualified, you'll no longer be able to contribute to your HSA, but you'll still be able to take money out of your HSA at any time in your life to pay for qualified medical expenses, with no taxes or penalties assessed. If you don't use the money for medical expenses and still have funds available after age sixty-five, you can withdraw them for non-medical purposes with no penalties, although income tax would be assessed at that point, with the HSA functioning much like a traditional IRA or 401(k).

A list of qualified medical expenses is available on the IRS website, www.irs.gov, in IRS Publication 502, "Medical and Dental Expenses."

Where Is My Account?

HSA bank accounts can be offered by your employer with easy payroll automatic deposit features, or you can set up an HSA account at one of the many participating banks throughout the country.

They are a great way to offset medical expenses on a pre-tax basis, and save tax-free for future medical or retirement expenses.

INDIVIDUAL PREMIUM TAX DEDUCTION

Additionally, if you're not on an employer plan, you don't qualify for subsidies under individual insurance and you itemize deductions on your tax returns, you can deduct qualified medical expenses that exceed 7.5 percent of your adjusted gross income for 2018. Beginning January 1, 2019, all taxpayers may deduct only the amount of the total unreimbursed allowable medical care expenses for the year that exceed 10 percent of their adjusted gross income. This includes health insurance premiums.

If you're self-employed and have a net profit for the year, you may be eligible for the self-employed health insurance deduction. This is an adjustment to income, rather than an itemized deduction, for premiums you paid on a health insurance policy covering medical care, including a qualified long-term care insurance policy covering medical care for yourself, your spouse, and dependents. In addition, you may be eligible for this deduction for your child who is under the age of twenty-seven at the end of 2017 even if the child wasn't your dependent. See chapter 6 of Publication 535, Business Expenses, for eligibility information. If you don't claim 100 percent of your paid premiums, you can include the remainder with your other medical expenses as an itemized deduction on Form 1040, Schedule A.pdf.[35]

Remember, you need to get professional tax advice on your specific situation.

LIFE EVENTS

Your life circumstances certainly affect how and when you attain health coverage. Let's look at a few scenarios.

---

35   Irs.gov. (2018). *Topic No. 502 Medical and Dental Expenses | Internal Revenue Service*. [online] Available at: https://www.irs.gov/taxtopics/tc502 [Accessed 24 Oct. 2018].

ENROLLING THROUGH YOUR EMPLOYER

Open enrollment is a period of time each year when you can sign up for health insurance. Employers' health plan open enrollments will vary by employer. Your employer will provide you with educational materials outlining the options and costs available to you. If you don't sign up for health insurance during open enrollment, you probably can't sign up for health insurance until the next open enrollment period, unless you experience a qualifying event.

If you're eligible and apply for health insurance during open enrollment, the health plan must insure you.

NEW HIRES

Non-seasonal new hires working thirty hours per week must be offered the employers' health plan within ninety days of starting the job. Your employer will provide you with information outlining your options as well as the corresponding features, costs, terms, and conditions.

Many employers now offer the open enrollment and/ or the new hire enrollment experience through online enrollment applications, but some still provide the information via paper materials.

INDIVIDUAL MARKETPLACE HEALTH INSURANCE

The open enrollment period for direct purchases of health insurance runs November 1 through December 15 with coverage effective January 1. You need to go through healthcare.gov or healthsherpa.com to qualify and receive subsidies, or through an insurance agent or directly with an insurance company if you do not qualify for a subsidy. Both websites provide benefit summaries and pricing for available coverage in your area. Similar to employer-sponsored health insurance, there may be some ways to enroll other than November 1 if you have a qualifying life event.

LEAVING YOUR EMPLOYER: DO YOU HAVE OPTIONS?

What happens to the healthcare plan you have if you leave your employer or lose employer benefits by moving to less than thirty hours of work with that employer? You can look at purchasing health insurance directly through the marketplace due to a qualifying life event (QLE), or continue to stay on your former employer's health plan extending your coverage due to the federal Consolidated Omnibus Budget Reconciliation Act, commonly known as COBRA. Upon terminating with your employer, voluntarily or involuntarily, you have sixty days to accept an offer to remain on your employer's plan for 102 percent of the full premium—your current monthly contribution plus the employer's contribution. You can maintain the coverage for eighteen months. Or, if you have dependents on the plan, they may remain for up to thirty-six months in the event of your death, divorce, or enrolling in Medicare. The coverage could be terminated if you fail to pay premiums timely, are eligible for another employer's group health plan, become entitled to Medicare, or commit fraud or perjury.

Staying on your employer's plan ensures continuity of what you have been used to. It's not cheap, but employer plans generally have broader provider networks and provide out-of-network benefits (if you're not in an HMO). You will want to see what's available in the marketplace, and whether you would qualify for a federal subsidy through ACA, and compare that to the COBRA option. Your employer is required to notify you of your COBRA rights and obligations at the time of your termination.

WHAT IF MY CIRCUMSTANCES CHANGE?

You can change your benefit elections whether you are on your employer plan or purchased individual insurance if you have experienced a qualifying life event (QLE). Qualifying life events include losing healthcare coverage, getting married/divorced, death of a covered member, having a baby, or adopting a child. A complete list can be found on healthcare.gov under QLE.

Sometimes, due to circumstances, you may face gaps in your coverage. What then? We'll cover that next.

CHAPTER TEN

ALTERNATIVE HEALTH PLANS, SUPPLEMENTAL HEALTH PLANS, AND CREATIVE FUNDING

President Trump enacted three regulatory provisions that will go into effect January 1, 2019, affecting the ACA and, therefore, you.

INDIVIDUAL MANDATE REPEAL

President Trump removed the individual mandate. You will no longer be charged a penalty if you don't have health insurance or have health insurance that is different from ACA coverage features. The intent was to allow people to consider plans that cover less and are less expensive to buy.[36]

SHORT-TERM, LIMITED-DURATION POLICIES

President Trump created regulations that allow the sale of short-term, limited-duration health insurance policies that offer less expensive coverage because they are not subject to ACA rules. The policies can cover you for up to one year. These policies have significant benefit limitations (most policies do not cover maternity services, limit prescription coverage, and do not offer substance abuse and mental illness treatment) and can restrict those who have an existing condition from getting coverage. People who developed a health problem would have covered services paid for but would not be renewed for the next year. At that point, they could reenter the ACA-compliant plans.

ASSOCIATION PLANS

President Trump created regulations that allow small employers and self-employed individuals to buy a new type of health plan that does not have to meet all ACA

---

36 Pollitz, Karen, and Gary Claxton. "Proposals for Insurance Options That Don't Comply with ACA Rules: Trade-offs In Cost and Regulation." The Henry J. Kaiser Family Foundation. August 20, 2018. Accessed September 26, 2018. https://www.kff.org/health-reform/issue-brief/proposals-for-insurance-options-that-dont-comply-with-aca-rules-trade-offs-in-cost-and-regulation/.

essential-benefit or pricing requirements. These plans could also screen for health conditions. Instead of buying health insurance individually, you now would be a member in a larger association and, thus, would be buying employer-style health insurance. The policies' premiums would be less expensive and could be a viable option for qualified participants. You will probably be contacted by trade associations if you are a member of associations for realtors, farmers, food service providers, janitors, or others.

> Do your homework. Know your health profile, study the exclusions, and understand what can happen to pricing at the annual renewal of the policy.

OTHER OPTIONS
INDIVIDUAL PROPRIETORS: HOW TO GET EMPLOYER OR GROUP INSURANCE

As I discussed, a large percentage of Americans are insured through their employer. With volume comes choice that we have previewed. We have also illustrated the many options available from carriers, covering plan designs to broader network options. We have also covered the individual market that is more restricted in all of those aforementioned options. You may be wondering: is there a way for an individual to play in the employer market versus the individual market? There may be.

Are you self-employed without any other employees buying health insurance through the individual market? If so, consider this: you are an employer. Most insurance carriers will not provide group insurance to one individual, but there may be other ways to approach the problem and access group (more flexible) insurance. Here are some examples to try:

- Look for affiliated trade associations. Inquire if they have a health plan and the requirements to join. President Trump passed an Executive Order that takes effect September 1, 2018, expanding the ability of associations to offer health insurance plans. Be careful to understand what they don't cover and if you can be excluded or experience reduced coverage for a preexisting condition.
- If an association health plan does not exist or fit your profile, consider aligning with other self-employed individuals and incorporating. Once you have two employees, you can contract with health insurance companies for employer-based coverage. This method would require legal and accounting costs not previously encountered, but it may be worth considering these days due to the high cost of individual health insurance and the limited options. If you go this route, more options open up to you, such as the following:
  ○ More flexible plans offering access to more health

insurance carriers and broader provider (hospitals and physician) networks.

- Chamber of commerce premium discounts, if a member.
- Access to employer-based healthcare benefits through a Professional Employer Organization (PEO). PEOs work with small businesses to help them manage payroll-related taxes, certain human resources functions, access to benefits, and other employer-related administrative functions necessary to running a business.

TIP

You want to work with an organization that has thousands of employees. You can google for PEOs in your area. Also, check with large national payroll companies; they have PEO divisions.

STUDENT COVERAGE

Many universities have phenomenal student coverage. They offer low-deductible, entirely comprehensive, ACA-compliant plans that can cover a student with low premiums. If you have a child in college and you're paying the family rate for insurance, consider taking your child off the family plan and enrolling in the university plan. Removing college student(s) from your current health insurance may allow you to drop from a family plan to a single plan or employee and spouse thus saving you premiums, and your child may have better benefits. Check with your child's college or university for available plans.

CHRISTIAN HEALTH PLANS

With the reduced carrier selections, increasing and sometimes unattainable premiums, and increased deductibles and coinsurance, people are aggressively looking for alternatives, any alternatives. Some are turning to nonprofit, religious-based plans, known as Christian healthcare plans, due to their significant reduction in premium costs and their exclusion from ACA penalties and requirements. These plans have seen tremendous growth over the past three years, paying close to two-thirds of a billion dollars in medical expenses and covering over 600,000 members in 2016.[37] Their explosive growth is eliciting greater interest and greater scrutiny. Both are warranted. Who are they? What do they offer? What don't they offer? What are their costs? Are they legitimate? Are they regulated? These and many more questions arise.

Christian health plans are healthcare-sharing ministries oriented toward practicing Christians. They are aligned with biblical teachings in that they hold believers have

---

37 "Home." Alliance of Health Care Sharing Ministries. Accessed April 19, 2018. http://www.healthcaresharing.org/.

a responsibility to assist each other's needs. They have been in existence for over twenty years and are growing rapidly due to their philosophy and low initial costs for healthcare solutions.

They are not insurance companies. They are excluded from ACA mandates like preexisting coverage exclusion, underwriting, and unlimited payments, due to their religious conviction. Members literally share in certain expenses covering one another's costs. Interestingly, this is the basic definition of insurance to aggregate expenses.

The major membership qualifications require: Christian testimony (live by biblical standards, bear one another's burdens, and regularly attend a fellowship of believers); healthy lifestyle (no smoking or illegal drugs); application review (underwriting—you can be denied for preexisting conditions); and health partners (be willing to participate with health coaches to work toward a healthier lifestyle). Interestingly again, this shared commitment to health produces solid aspects of the program that work in improving the members' lives and keeping health costs in control, thereby leading to better quality of life for the individual.

Some Christian health plans have PPO network providers, and some don't. All encourage you to negotiate fees with providers and have provider counselors to assist with negotiations if providers refuse. By stating they aren't insurance and are paying cash, the members are generally successfully receiving significant discounts off of the published provider charges—a phenomenon we will discuss in a later chapter on negotiation. The programs have annual contributions that grant you "sharing" amounts per qualified illness. Each illness will require a deductible from you before the illness is submitted for sharing. Non-qualified or preexisting condition bills can be submitted as financial prayer requests that may or may not be met by the membership. Each individual is assessed on the annual contribution level and then will also receive financial prayer requests from others throughout the year. Most of the entry-level plans do not cover prescription drugs. Gold plans often do.

When considering these plans, or any other plan for that matter, do not just read the covered procedures. Find the exclusion section, generally in the appendix of their coverage guide, and scrutinize those features. Make sure your health profile, which includes your family health history, does not include those features. Common exclusions with these plans are preexisting illnesses, prescription medicine, chiropractic treatments, diagnostic services, birth control, and illegal drug-related services.

The healthcare-sharing ministry landscape is dominated by five major players with the largest memberships and highest revenue spread across the country and across Christian denominations. Samaritan Ministries (in Illinois), Christian Healthcare Ministries (in Ohio), and Medishare (in Florida) are the three large evangelical operations. Dozens of similar ministries exist across the country, mostly smaller and more localized. Ohio's Liberty HealthShare is Mennonite, a denomination traditionally committed to pacifism and dialogue. Solidarity HealthShare, founded in 2015, is Catholic, and partnered with another Mennonite aid group in Ohio to be grandfathered into the ACA exemption for sharing ministries, which required that they exist before 1999. There is also a Jewish-based health plan found at unitedrefuahhs.org.

If you're interested in one of these plans, analyze the plan designs, rules, and regulations. Seek out current participants who have had large claims. Find out what worked for them and what didn't, and go from there.

SUPPLEMENTAL HEALTH PLANS

You've just purchased a health policy and had to increase the deductibles and out-of-pocket costs to afford the monthly premium. You're not sure where you're going to come up with the money, but you felt like you had no alternative based on the costs of the lower-deductible plans. Sure, your insurance will kick in after you meet that deductible, but what do you do if you can't meet your deductible in the first place? When shopping for insurance, it's easy to overlook that deductibles represent real money out of your pocket. Your grocery bills, mortgages, and car payments don't stop just because you have a medical expense you need to cover. In this chapter, we'll talk about filling in those gaps in coverage with alternative funding options.

These are not healthcare policies and should not be considered as a replacement of an ACA-qualified health plan. They may make sense, depending on your budget and health concerns, to offset the effects of a catastrophic illness on your finances. You'll wonder, "Where do I get the money to cover the deductibles and out-of-pocket costs of my insurance plan caused by medical expenses? If I'm not working because I'm sick, how do I cover those costs?"

Supplemental policies offer you direct cash payment in the event you have a critical illness, hospital stay, or accident. They can be purchased directly from the insurance carriers or agents and are often offered through your employer. Programs can be designed to meet your specific needs and affordability, and they can provide peace of mind. They are not reduced or coordinated with other health insurance you own and are generally extremely affordable—usually under $50 a month. Supplemental policies have become increasingly popular due to the escalating premium costs that have driven most of us to higher-deductible plans. If you have a lower out-of-pocket healthcare plan, note that you likely don't need a supplemental plan. In other words, if your deductible is $500, why would you buy a $5,000 cancer policy? The direct payments can be purchased at different levels, allowing you to fit them to your specific needs. Underwriting requirements are nominal for basic levels of coverage. Preexisting exclusions do apply to individuals with an existing condition. There are basically three types of coverage: critical illness, accident and hospital, and medical indemnity plans. We will briefly cover what each entails, what to watch for, who the players are, and where to get it.[38]

CRITICAL ILLNESS

Critical illness covers expenses resulting from specific diseases. The benefit amount is paid in a lump-sum payment when you are diagnosed with that named disease. The most common illnesses covered are as follows:

· Heart Attack
· Cancer
· Stroke
· Organ Transplant

---

38 If you have an HSA plan, you're probably better off saving the premiums to offset of pocket costs versus buying these products. Remember, the dollars you save in the HSA are *your money* and will grow if not used. Premiums for these products are gone once you spend them, and you may or may not have any claims.

- Heart Transplant
- Kidney Failure
- Coronary Bypass Surgery
- Paralysis
- And more

You can purchase coverage amounts as low as $5,000 per disease up to $50,000 by answering basic health questions. Amounts over $50,000 require full medical underwriting. Costs range from $50/month to $150/month depending on your age and the coverage amount selected.

ACCIDENT COVERAGE

Accident and health coverage simply means plans that pay covered expenses related to accidents. They're paid in a lump-sum payment to you to use as you deem appropriate and are not limited to, or coordinated with, other medical coverage you have. Covered conditions can include the following as long as they are due to an accident:

- Fractures
- Dislocations
- Concussions
- Lacerations
- Second- and Third-Degree Burns
- Ruptured Discs

- Torn Knee Cartilage
- And more

HOSPITAL INDEMNITY

Hospital indemnity covers expenses for hospital admissions, allowing a daily rate up to a maximum number of days and dollars. You can purchase daily benefits of $100–$1,000 per day for a period of up to 180 consecutive days. Coverage for the following is included under this type of plan:

- Intensive Care Units
- Emergency Room Visits
- Qualifying Outpatient Visits
- And more

THE SUPPLEMENTAL MARKET: WHAT YOU NEED TO KNOW

Plans like those I've described are becoming more popular as deductibles and out-of-pocket costs rise. So, more insurance companies are now offering those plans. Newcomers in the field are the major health carriers—Aetna, Cigna, Humana, Blue Cross Blue Shield, and United Healthcare—which are now offering the coverages in addition to their comprehensive, ACA-compliant health insurance offerings.

The following companies, on the other hand, have been

offering these coverages for decades: Aflac, Mutual of Omaha, Colonial Life Insurance Company, Principal Financial Group, Assurity Life Insurance, Co-American Fidelity, Assurance, Guardian Life Insurance Company of America, Assurant Health Company, Combined Insurance, and AIG.

Critical illness, accident and hospital, and medical indemnity coverages should be considered when creating your total healthcare insurance package. You may be able to select a higher-deductible health plan at a lower premium and purchase one of these programs for less than the cost of buying a lower-deductible health plan. Note: these options don't cover medical expenses (like pharmacy expenses) but they do offset catastrophic expenses.

TIP: DON'T OVERINSURE YOURSELF

Only buy the amount of coverage that covers your deductible and out-of-pocket expenses before your health insurance plan pays 100 percent. Only purchase the plan if one of these plans and your health insurance plan combined *is less than a lower-deductible health insurance plan*. Otherwise, you are overinsured.

CREATIVE FUNDING SOLUTIONS

If you are in a dire situation and need money to offset medical bills, here are some suggestions to untap cash.

LIFE INSURANCE OPTIONS

Another feature to be keenly aware of when purchasing life insurance is an advance benefit rider. An advanced benefit rider offers you access to the face amount (the amount of life insurance you are covered for) while you are alive—and tax-free! They apply to people diagnosed with terminal illnesses who need to cover long-term care expenses. Check to see if your current policy has this feature.

If you're trying to determine whether or not to purchase life insurance to cover long-term care expenses, remember that it's a different world now. Looking at life insurance through a new lens might make sense. First of all, it still provides a death benefit. Now with cash value and the ability to sell policies, life insurance takes on a whole new function in your financial planning. For example, term insurance with advanced benefits is relatively inexpensive into your forties. Check with a financial or life insurance advisor.

OTHER FUNDING SOLUTIONS

- Ask for a payment plan. Once a provider knows you're willing to pay the tab, they should work with you. Ask your hospital, too. Many have charitable plans or financial assistance plans.
- Look for assistance from disease-based medical associations, religions, and medical charity groups. Do your research. There are generally three categories to search: disease-specific organizations (cancer, heart, kidney, etc.); religious organizations (Christian denominations, Jewish, Islamic, etc.); and general charities specializing in medical financial assistance. They are out there. The assistance they provide ranges from health insurance premium assistance to assisting with copays, deductibles, and out-of-pocket costs. Ask for help. For example, the American Kidney Fund Health Insurance Premium Program (HIPP) has been known to pay the insurance premiums of patients on kidney dialysis as they wait for transplants, which can sometimes take years. Again, their assistance is not guaranteed, but the least you can do is ask. The worst they can say is no, and you'll be in the same position you were in before. You can't be afraid to ask for help, especially when your health is on the line. Here's a sampling of organizations that provide financial assistance:
  - Patient Access Network Foundation (1-866-316-7263)

- Patient Services, Inc. (1-800-366-7741)
- HealthWellFoundation (1-800-675-8416)
- The Leukemia & Lymphoma Society's patient financial aid program (1-800-955-4572)
- Cancer*Care* (1-800-813-4673)
- Patient Access Network (PAN)
- Religious charities: check with your church, mosque, or temple to see what assistance they lend or if they're affiliated with any entity that can help.

· Dedicate a credit card to medical expenses. If you're like me, you get more credit card offers in the mail than you can shake a stick at. Take one, put it in a drawer, and don't touch it. If you run into a catastrophe and need access to $5,000 to pay a deductible, you can pull the card out, activate it, and use the money. Yes, you'll have to pay the horrible 15 to 20 percent interest rates, but at least you'll receive your healthcare. If you can, apply for a credit limit that covers your total out-of-pocket costs associated with your health insurance plan. Think of this option as emergency insurance on your insurance. And note, I'd only suggest this credit card trick in the case of a true emergency, as it does come with a hefty side of risk. Still, it can be effective if you're struggling.

· Take out a home equity loan. A home equity loan can provide the same cash as a credit card, with one caveat: you have to borrow the money before you need it. If you try to take out a loan with a $5,000 bill, the bank won't lend you the money. This is one more reason why you should always be aware of your healthcare situation, so you're more likely to be able to spot potential trouble before you find yourself in the financial weeds.

- Utilize your employer tax-savings plans. Many employers will offer Section 125, HSA, or FSA programs. Section 125 plans allow you to take pretaxed deductions from your retirement account to help you pay for insurance premiums or healthcare bills. For example, if you get taxed at 30 percent for your income, a Section 125 plan allows you to put 100 percent of your gross take home pay—before it's taxed—toward your premiums. It's like getting a 17 to 30 percent discount on premiums—it's a no-brainer. Rather than putting that pretaxed money toward premiums, an HSA builds it up into an account, which can be used to pay for medical bills, dental bills, and money toward your deductible. FSA programs are another way to save for medical expenses, but the difference is the money disappears at the end of the year. If you don't use it, you lose it! If you get access to any of these programs from your employer, take them. You're only increasing the utility of your dollar.
- Set up a GoFundMe campaign. Every day, there are more GoFundMe campaigns hitting the internet for various reasons, many of them medical. An associate

had a family member get cancer, and they couldn't cover the deductible. As a last resort, they set up a GoFundMe page and raised $15,000. The process is not guaranteed, in a way similar to the church programs I discussed earlier, and relies on the goodness of other people to be successful.

· Tap into any life insurance policies you own. Term plans can help with raising cash. Life settlement companies, for instance, will buy your term insurance from you. They pay you a fraction of the death benefit. Whole life policies, on the other hand, present more options. Your policy builds cash value accounts over time. Many forget or don't understand they can borrow that money. You may have access to cash to pay large, unforeseen medical charges and out-of-pocket costs!

CASE IN POINT

An older acquaintance of mine was diagnosed with a serious chronic condition and was worried that he and his spouse's income sources would not be sufficient to cover the growing medical costs. Interestingly enough, he'd had long-standing whole life insurance policies for years—the cash value of which exceeded over $100,000. In his mind, those policies were bought for death benefits, and he had discounted his ability to access the cash for other purposes (i.e., his health expenses). Refamiliarizing himself with this revelation eased his financial anxiety.

The point of these alternative methods is to transfer risk. I'm not naïve—I know that once you take out $5,000 on a credit card or sell your life insurance or use the equity on your house to pay medical bills, you'll have to pay back that money. **But you remove the debilitating financial stress and can focus on managing your health.**

You know yourself, your risk, and all the nitty gritty details about how to choose and finance the right plan for you. Now, let's take a deeper dive into what it truly means to be a healthcare consumer. Let's first explore how we educate and empower ourselves with the essence of the issue, cost, and the outcome of our healthcare services.

PART III

NAVIGATING HEALTHCARE: BECOME A SMART CONSUMER

CHAPTER ELEVEN

FINDING THE RIGHT PROVIDER

At some point in your life, you're going to need to select a medical provider. Maybe you're starting a family and you need an OBGYN. Maybe you've been diagnosed with a specific condition and you need a specialist. Maybe you aren't happy with your current level of care and are seeking a new primary care physician. In these instances, and so many more, one question comes up: How do you choose the right provider? The insurance companies can't decide for you. Ultimately, it's your decision, and I'm going to guide you through how to make the best choice.

CONSIDER THIS

Kara Trott, founder and CEO of Quantum Health, conducted a two-year consumer behavioral study that tracked the healthcare journey of 3,200 consumers, with 290 physicians participating. The focus of the study was to map out each journey. An unexpected finding of the study was how critical the starting point of the journey was. They found that 41 percent of the consumers self-referred to a physician, and 61 percent of those self-referrals were to the wrong physician—a dynamic that resulted in a 33 percent higher cost and a delay in receiving treatment.[39]

Those increased costs come in the form of wasted time and potentially incorrect diagnoses. This data shows it's important for your physical health and financial health that you find the right doctor who will know you and help you.

WHERE DO I START?

Looking at the list of possible healthcare providers is like wading through a sea of names, organizations, specialties, and affiliations. It can be daunting. You may

---

39 The Business of Transforming Healthcare: The Consumer's Journey: Trott on Trends in Healthcare." https://quantum-health.com/News-Events/Downloads/Quantum-Health-The-Consumers-Journey-112316.pdf.

wonder, "Where do I start? Who's right for me and my situation? They're all doctors, right?" (Remember the joke about what you call the person who finished last in medical school? A doctor!) You might wonder, "Does it even matter who I choose, anyway? Can't I just go with the doctor at the top of the list?"

My response? You *could*, yes. But do I recommend that approach? No! Instead, why don't we apply the approaches we've adopted in creating our health profile to selecting our caregivers and see what different results we can achieve? Let's start at your home base: your primary care doctor.

General practitioners and primary care physicians are gatekeepers to the medical community. They are the first people to diagnose your conditions and provide you with a broader perspective based on your personal history. As they get to know you, they will be able to diagnose you more effectively. They are the ones who make your referrals to specialists they know and trust.

You need a personal relationship with your primary care physician. When you enter the confusing world of healthcare, you need an advocate on your side, someone who knows your personal health history and can diagnose you appropriately. Your physician should also be able to navigate you through the system when you encounter a problem beyond their expertise. It is incredibly important to select a primary care physician wisely because it's the choice that will impact your experience throughout the entire healthcare system. Their referrals also grant you enhanced access to specialists. Without them, you may not get an appointment, or you may have longer waiting times.

YOU AREN'T YOUR OWN DOCTOR

Be careful not to play doctor yourself. Yes, you need to understand your own health, but be wary of simply searching your symptoms on WebMD and visiting your primary care doctor with a self-diagnosis. Your goal is to use transparency tools to understand more about your own conditions, who is qualified to treat them, and who is the most cost effective. That way, as a more informed consumer, you can find someone who can help steer you in the direction of the right specialists.

Many people will self-refer to a specialist. Often times, they choose that provider for the wrong reasons, such as a review on a website. The information on some review sites is not complete. Reviewers will often talk about factors like waiting room time and how friendly the physician was in person. That's all well and good—and it is part of the equation—but you need more. You need to understand their experience, common outcomes, and pricing. Those qualities are the difference-makers in a specialist. A good primary care doctor knows you and your medical needs and the medical community. They are best suited to guide you to effective medical care.

Everything is a balance. If you find a doctor who is too kind, they might not motivate you to take control of your own health. If a doctor is too harsh, you might shy away from going to them and only exacerbate your problems. You won't know who is exactly right for you unless you do some experimenting. Remember, though, not to play doctor for yourself. Ask questions and be selective on what advice you follow.

HOW TO CHOOSE A DOCTOR

First things first: you need to establish a relationship with a primary doctor and/or an OBGYN. If you don't know where to start when searching for a primary care doctor, start with referrals from other doctors, your community, or your workplace. If you are new to an area, the local hospitals may provide you with a referral. Understand, though, that the hospital will point you toward one of their own doctors. Once you gather a name, or multiple names, do your research through the transparency tools we have highlighted: Guroo, Amino Health, Healthcare Bluebook, Vitals, Healthgrades, AMA, and Doctorfinder are examples. You may need to utilize a combination of tools comparing ones that offer information about the practice: waiting times, ease of working with, length of time in business, outcome, cost-based information, and more. As you develop a list of possible candidates, check your insurance carrier's "in-network" physician directory to ensure your selections are on the list. The health insurance directories should promote the most cost-effective ones and know who is accepting new patients.

When searching for the right primary care doctor, there are a number of factors to consider, for example:

- How easy are they to access?
- What is the quality of their care?
- What do they charge?
- Are they in your network or out of it?
- Are they board certified?
- Do they have experience managing your condition(s)?
- How long have they been in business?
- Are they taking new patients?
- What is their hospital affiliation?
- Are there any red flags such as malpractice suits or sanctions?
- Are they vested in technology?
- Do they participate in electronic medical records and coordinate electronically with pharmacists, other specialists, hospitals, and you?

Once you start to sort through potential doctors based on these questions and select one, use your first visit to continue your research. What is your compatibility with the doctor? Do they listen to you? Do they communicate effectively by outlining the purpose of your visit and help you both come to conclusions together, rather than just dictating them to you? Is their staff friendly, efficient, and respectful? Do they get the doctor your messages in a timely manner and address insurance concerns? Your doctor should make you feel comfortable and confident—more like a partner in your healthcare journey.

One way to cut through the clutter is to ask if the practice is a participating Patient Centered Medical Homes, or PCMH, practice. PCMH is a byproduct of ACA. PCMH certification requires physicians to have certain features and services offered for their patients. PCMHs work to lower the fragmentation in the healthcare system by encouraging effective communication among providers and by not duplicating medical records and tests. They do everything electronically, all with the aim of improving the quality of healthcare, reducing costs, and improving the patient experience. They look at doctors' offices and tell them they have to operate more like a business in an effort to make sure staff is happy, patients are happy, and their information is up-to-date. If you find a doctor is who PCMH-certified, you know they've proactively taken steps to be more efficient and focused on your happiness.

At the end of the day, your primary doctor should understand where you are, value your time, and respect you as a person. Your doctor will make decisions *with* you, not for you, so they need to be someone who actively listens and looks at the big picture. They also need to keep money in mind. They should tell you what everything means in a language you can understand. They should be transparent, which means they give you access to your records. They should encourage you to bring help if you need it, and they should see your care as a learning process between the two of you. If you choose correctly, your doctor won't bite when you ask questions—even tough ones.

Selecting a specialist is where your hard work in partnering with the right primary care physician pays off. If and when you need a specialist, your PCP is the best person for the job. You should have developed a clinical and personal relationship with them that allows them to effectively direct your care. Their informed referrals grant you access to the specialist community on a timely basis; their recommendations and referrals should be given heavy consideration.

That doesn't mean you should solely rely on your primary care doctor's referral. Supplement it with your own research, utilizing one of the listed transparency sites that compares costs, outcomes, and the volume of procedures that the specialist performs per year. The sites analyze billions of medical claims and can report on the number of procedures a specialist has performed and at what cost. This allows them to predict the top performers among their peer set across the country. Then, it will show you how their procedure volume ranks against doctors across the country.

This level of research is important because, while doctors aren't perfect, you want to find someone who has years of practice without years' worth of mistakes. In his book *Outliers*, Malcolm Gladwell says that you need 10,000 hours of practice in anything to become an expert. If you find a doctor or specialist who has done more procedures and seen more patients, they're probably the better doctor. Remember: volume is everything when selecting a specialist!

MY SURGICAL MISTAKE

When I had hip surgery, I chose the wrong specialist. My primary care doctor referred me to a hip surgeon who had zero personality, was not interested in my research and experiences related to my hip, and had a "take it or leave it" attitude. I didn't like him, so I interviewed three more surgeons and found someone whom I had a better rapport with. Even though he was proficient, he didn't have as many surgeries under his belt as the arrogant doctor.

In the end, I was less than pleased with the result of my surgery. In retrospect, I should have taken a different approach to choosing my specialist. A specialist, like a hip surgeon, is not there to coddle you and create a long-term relationship with you. They are there to provide you with good care for a specific situation. Unlike your primary care physician, you're not there for a holistic approach. Your relationship is confined to that specific procedure. My primary care doctor knew this, and I should have listened to him. Again, volume is king.

Note: if your condition is chronic and requires a specialist, you will develop the same partnership relationship you have with your primary physician.

Finding the right physician team is like everything else: it takes time and effort. It also has a lot to do with (also like everything else) whom you know. Thankfully, the world of transparency is allowing us to look under the hood more than we have ever been able to before. This only enhances our decision process and ultimate selections.

NONTRADITIONAL PROVIDER OPTIONS

Not everyone approaches healthcare the same way. Cost of care, higher out-of-pocket costs, technology, and transparency are all causing the medical field to evolve. The evolution is producing nontraditional provider options. Let's look at a few.

TELEMEDICINE

In chapter 7, I listed telemedicine as an additional service provided by most insurance providers. Here, let's examine telemedicine in depth, not as an extra service but as a nontraditional provider of regular services. Telemedicine offers medical consultations over the phone, Skype, or FaceTime, and it's a piece of the healthcare industry that is constantly growing. In fact, the global telehealth market is projected to reach 12.1 billion by 2023, with a compound annual growth rate of 23 percent between 2018 and 2023.[40]

With fewer doctors able to give significant time to patients, telemedicine can serve as the front line of medicine. In addition, rural areas yearn for good medical care, so teledoctors are a great way to provide service to people who can't easily get in to a doctor. One of the advancements in services that is propelling telemedicine is the ability to prescribe medicine through their service. Some services can refer to specialists and facilitate the scheduling of the specialist's appointment.

---

40   "$12.1 Billion Telehealth/Telemedicine Market: 2018-2023 Global Analysis &
       Forecast Report - ResearchAndMarkets.com." Business Wire. July 27, 2018. Accessed
       September 26, 2018. https://www.businesswire.com/news/home/20180727005463/
       en/12.1-Billion-TelehealthTelemedicine-Market-2018-2023-Global-Analysis.

Another plus: teledoctor visits are usually discounted compared to traditional in-office visits. If a doctor visit costs approximately $100 on your plan, a telemedicine "visit" might only be $49. Even if your carrier doesn't offer a telemedicine service, you can buy it directly from some hospitals such as the Cleveland Clinic and Premier Hospital in Dayton, Ohio, or from Teladoc—that's what makes it more than just an insurance bonus! You don't even have to be in their area to use the service. In addition, Walgreens recently cut a deal with New York Presbyterian to provide telemedicine in the greater New York area. There's a movement to give people quality, non-emergency healthcare through flexible, timesaving access to doctors. Telemedicine is the private market responding to the market needs. Using technology, we are reinstating the doctor "house calls." It's worth considering twenty-four-hour care in your home with qualified practitioners at a fraction of the cost!

Laura, whom I interviewed for this book, was skeptical that anything anyone could say would reduce the healthcare deck stacked against her. She relayed her recent story of frustration, anger, and anxiety over the healthcare and health insurance industry. She and her family, like most of us, lived on a fixed budget and had to elect a high-deductible plan due to rising premiums. Her young daughter woke up in the middle of the night on a weekend complaining of an earache. She had a high fever as well. Her pediatrician did not have after-hours weekend services, and the answering service was not responding quickly. So, she took her daughter to the emergency room. The diagnosis? An ear infection. The treatment? Antibiotics. The total cost of both? Over $300 which she had to pay because of her high-deductible plan. I then told her about a better option: telemedicine.

CLINICS

What do Wal-Mart, Safeway, Kroger, Target, Walgreens, and CVS all have in common? They all offer health clinics within their select stores. More and more, traditional retailers are bringing their retail expertise to medicine to provide easier-access, lower-cost alternatives to healthcare.

The clinics provide services similar to a primary care doctor and are staffed by registered nurses (RNs), nurse practitioners (NPs), and physician assistants (PAs). Services include treating minor illnesses; screening for and monitoring minor injuries, handling skin conditions, conducting wellness exams and physicals, performing women's services, and giving vaccinations and injections. They diagnose, treat, and prescribe medicines at a lower cost. Fees range from $49-$99 and are accepted by most insurance carriers. Check on their websites for locations that have a clinic and for insurance carriers that accept their services.

TIP

If prescribed medicine at one of the pharmacy companies' clinics, make sure you are getting the best price on the prescription before filling it.

CONCIERGE SERVICES: CUTTING THROUGH THE CLUTTER

Most primary care practices are inundated with patients, ranging from two thousand to three thousand per physician. They typically see twenty to twenty-four patients a day—a rate that equates to spending an average of eight minutes with each patient (after you take into account paperwork, lunch, and breaks). Does eight minutes seem like enough time to develop a holistic approach to you? No, it doesn't, and many physicians don't think so either. As a result, they have been morphing their practices into concierge service providers; in fact, there were over 12,000 in 2014.[41]

A concierge practice charges an annual retainer, generally $1,500 per year, waives your insurance copay or deductible for office visits, and submits claims for services to your carrier. Most concierge practices are primary care or general internist doctors. They limit their practice to 400–600 patients per year, allowing them to extend their

---

41   Dalen, J. and Alpert, J. (2018). *Concierge Medicine Is Here and Growing!!*. [online] Available at: https://www.amjmed.com/article/S0002-9343(17)30358-3/fulltext [Accessed 21 Sep. 2018].

time with each patient. You may be wondering why you would want to spend an additional $1,500 per year on top of your insurance to see your doctor? The answer is simple: enhanced service and access. Concierge practices offer immediate access to their doctors via cell phone, email, and same-day appointments. Visits are, on average, thirty minutes, granting time to cover all issues. Additional attention is provided with referrals to specialists or hospitals, and some services offer home or hospital visits as well as access to top specialists.

In short, they're the clinical advocates they once were, but at an additional cost. Most practices are located in or near large cities and on the coasts. Two national practices are MDVIP and Pinnacle.

MEDICAL TOURISM

Rather than staying in the US, some people seek healthcare outside their area—whether internationally or domestically—in order to save money. This process is known as medical tourism, and it started to gain traction even before the ACA came along. People who don't have coverage or are underinsured might need medical procedures but can't pay for them out-of-pocket, for example, so they seek out cheaper care beyond where they live. This can either be in other areas in the US or internationally.

US TOURISM

The cost of medical services varies widely in the US, and higher cost doesn't always mean better outcomes. We have already explored the hospital markups in the US, and you know certain areas have higher markups and that costs vary greatly from hospital to hospital.

The following information, directly from Blue Cross and Blue Shield, provides a glimpse into this issue:[42]

"A Study of Cost Variations for Knee and Hip Replacement Surgeries in the U.S." shows the average typical cost (without complications, see footnote) for a total knee replacement procedure was $31,124 in 64 markets where claims data was reviewed. However, it could cost as little as $11,317 in Montgomery, Alabama, and as much as $69,654 in New York, New York. Within a market, extreme cost variation can also exist. In Dallas, Texas, a total knee replacement could cost between $16,772 and $61,585 (267 percent cost variation) depending on the hospital.

Similar trends were also seen for the average typical cost for a total hip replacement procedure, which averaged $30,124. However, the procedure could cost as little

---

42   Bcbs.com. (2018). *Blue Cross Blue Shield Association Study Reveals Extreme Cost Variations for Knee and Hip Replacement Surgeries | Blue Cross Blue Shield*. [online] Available at: https://www.bcbs.com/news/press-releases/blue-cross-blue-shield-association-study-reveals-extreme-cost-variations-knee [Accessed 21 Sep. 2018].

as $11,327 in Birmingham, Alabama, and as much as $73,987 in Boston, Massachusetts, which had the greatest variance within a market, with costs as low as $17,910 (313 percent cost variation).

Additionally, certain hospitals have superior outcomes for diseases they specialize in. To that end, many insurance plans offer Centers of Excellence programs where they encourage members to consider selected healthcare experts in their field across the country in order to secure better outcomes and better pricing—a win-win for everyone. Check your program to see if they are offered in your plan. If not, use some of the transparency tools that we have highlighted and do your own research. The extra effort might surprise you.

CASE STUDIES IN FRUGALITY

A gentleman in northern Michigan was looking at the cheapest MRI in his town at $1,300. He researched through his carrier, Blue Cross Blue Shield of Michigan, and found the same service in a city three hours away at $600. He had a $5,000 deductible. He made the trip. As another example, research with Guroo shows that an average knee replacement in San Francisco is $61,817 and $30,726 in Phoenix.

Further cost savings are available outside the US and might provide quality care for as low as 15 percent of what it would cost in America. Even including airfare and hotels, it's cheaper for some patients to make trips overseas in search of treatment rather than foot the bill to have that same treatment here. It's important to note that medical tourism doesn't make sense for all ailments; it's mostly good for dental care, orthopedic replacements, gastric bypasses, stomach stapling, and cosmetics surgeries, or if you are uninsured or underinsured and want to explore less costly options.

As time goes on, medical tourism is going to evolve and become more prominent. About 1.4 million Americans per year use medical tourism to save money. Savings vary by procedure and country. How much can you save? Here's a listing highlighting the percentage reduction in healthcare countries' medical costs versus US costs across a variety of specialties and procedures for the most traveled destinations, courtesy of Patients Beyond Borders:[43]

- Brazil: 20–30 percent
- Costa Rica: 45–65 percent

---

43 Patientsbeyondborders.com. (2018). *Patients Beyond Borders | The most trusted resource in medical travel.* [online] Available at: https://patientsbeyondborders.com/ [Accessed 21 Sep. 2018].

- India: 65-90 percent
- Malaysia: 65-80 percent
- Mexico: 40-65 percent
- Singapore: 25-40 percent
- South Korea: 30-45 percent
- Taiwan: 40-55 percent
- Thailand: 50-75 percent
- Turkey: 50-65 percent

How do you know where to go for which procedures? Patients Beyond Borders is a wonderful resource if you're interested in learning more about specific procedures and countries.

13 QUESTIONS TO ASK WHEN YOU CONSIDER MEDICAL TOURISM

According to Patients Beyond Borders, if you are going to consider international medical tourism, be sure to have the following questions satisfactorily answered.[44]

1. Is the country itself safe?
2. If the healthcare costs are incredibly cheap, are they still of high quality?
3. What are the surgeon's qualifications?
4. How much exactly will you be saving?

---

44 "The Most Trusted Resource in Medical Travel." Patients Beyond Borders. Accessed September 26, 2018. https://patientsbeyondborders.com/.

5. What treatments do they have available in the country?

6. Can I easily access the area with cheap treatments?

7. Once I receive medical attention, how long will it take me to recover and come home?

8. Do they speak English?

9. What happens if I encounter complications after I've come home?

10. Does my health insurance cover my overseas expenses?

11. Can I sue the healthcare provider?

12. What recourses do I have if something goes wrong?

13. Will they allow me to finance my treatment?

Now you know how to find the right doctor for you, and you've learned what types of nontraditional options are available. Once you have vetted your options and have chosen a provider, how do you form a relationship with them?

The process is simple, yet not easy. Let me explain.

CHAPTER TWELVE

DEVELOPING A WINNING RELATIONSHIP

You've researched, been referred, and reached out to schedule an appointment with your chosen primary care physician. How do you get the most out of this relationship? Remember, your doctor is the clinician who should know you best and holistically.

They make the primary diagnosis. They are the ones who will cut through the healthcare system clutter and ease your way into the best appropriate specialties and hospitals. They will even help you save money. Developing a good, solid relationship with this person is the best start or foundation of your healthcare experience. Your doctor is your teammate and advocate. And no, this isn't a fantasy; it can be a reality, and one you can achieve without bribing your physician with candy, flowers, or a bottle of Maker's Mark. If you're educating yourself, being proactive about your health, and providing the right information, you can establish the kind of relationship that is healthy for you both physically and financially.

The process is like any other valuable relationship you have: simple if you approach it with the right mindset and effort, but not necessarily what we have traditionally done with our healthcare professionals. The keys to success are preparation, clear two-way communication, and clear goals. Remember, you've got an average of eight minutes per visit with the doctor. Your goal is to efficiently communicate to the doctor your ailments and expectations.[45] Let's review some tips on how to maximize that experience and develop a relationship with your doctor.

PREPARATION

Be organized. Studies have shown that patients who filled out a detailed checklist asked more questions during their doctor visit and got more satisfaction with the visit. The checklist should include accurate information, dates, times, and circumstances about your symptoms, your health record you developed in chapter 3 (including any

---

45 Stephen Permut, MD, chairman, family and community medicine, Temple University School of Medicine, Philadelphia. Kinnersley, P. *Cochrane Database of Systematic Reviews*, July 18, 2007; Issue 3. Terrie Wurzbacher, MD, author, *Your Doctor Said What? Exposing the Communication Gap*.

and all medications you are taking), and a list of questions you wish to cover. Prioritize the questions to three or four in order of importance to you.

CONFIDENT COMMUNICATION WITH YOUR HEALTHCARE PROVIDER

Read this sentence twice to truly get it in your head: it's your responsibility to communicate effectively with your doctor. You have to be organized when it comes to your own health. Stephen Covey wrote that to effectively communicate, both parties have to "seek first to understand and then to be understood." Understanding the doctor's environment sets you up to further prepare your discussion with them. What better way to prepare is there than understanding how they are trained to communicate with themselves? Many physician practices and hospitals use a technique called SBAR (Situation Background Assessment Recommendation). It was developed by the Navy for use in nuclear submarines to enhance efficient communication. Staff and physicians use SBAR to share patient information in a clear, complete, concise, and structured format and to improve communication, efficiency, and accuracy. Here's the framework and how it relates to you:

- Situation: Take ten seconds to explain (your aliment reason for the appointment)

- Background: Provide context and data (your medical health record)
- Assessment: Describe the specific problem/situation (doctor's diagnosis)
- Recommendation: Explain what you want to do about it and when (course of treatment)

Try not to get emotional or engage in non-essential stories. Stick with the facts! Also, don't withhold information on embarrassing symptoms, issues, or cost concerns that are causing fear. Without that information, the doctor can't help you. By being prepared and fact-based, the two of you will have more time to focus on your issues and questions. You have to be concise, organized, objective, and precise.

COMMUNICATION CONSEQUENCES

The more thorough you are, the more you can save yourself from later complications. John, a plastic surgeon, once was prepping someone to go under anesthetic before surgery when the patient suddenly revealed she had been taking a particular medication. John knew the drug she mentioned did not mix with anesthesia, and it would have created serious complications in surgery. He stopped the entire procedure. The patient wasn't pleased. Had he proceeded, the patient would have been in danger. The irony would have been had he proceeded without that knowledge and negative complications arose, he would have faced a lawsuit! The lesson? You're not doing yourself any favors when you withhold or forget to include information, so always err on the side of being thorough. Your health is in your hands.

TIP

Take an advocate with you to the appointment who can make sure you cover your situation and key questions. They can also be another set of ears to listen to the doctor's diagnosis and course of treatment. Take notes during the appointment and ask for a summary of the appointment from your doctor outlining their diagnosis and treatment plan. This can often be accessed online as well.

Looking for some assistance in developing good questions to ask your doctor? The US Agency for Healthcare Research and Quality (AHRQ), a division of the Department of Health and Human Services, has included on its website (ahrq.gov/patients-consumers/patient-involvement/ask-your-doctor/index.html) a "tips and tools" section on what to do before during and after your appointment. Sample questions are:

· What is the test for?
· How many times have you done this procedure?

- When will I get the results?
- Why do I need this treatment?
- Are there any alternatives?
- What are the possible complications?
- Which hospital is best for my needs?
- How do you spell the name of that drug?
- Are there any side effects?
- Will this medicine interact with medicines that I'm already taking?
- What is my diagnosis?
- What are my treatment options? What are the benefits of each option? What are the side effects?
- Will I need a test? What is the test for? What will the results tell me?
- What will the medicine you are prescribing do? How do I take it? Are there any side effects?
- Why do I need surgery? Are there other ways to treat my condition? How often do you perform this surgery?
- Do I need to change my daily routine?

EXTREME STORY

Martha, whose daughter has an undiagnosed seizure disorder, taught me about the SBAR technique. As a result of the debilitating medical condition, her daughter was on a feeding tube and couldn't speak. Because the child's situation was so rare, Martha had to become the advocate for her daughter. In this case, the internet became a glorious healthcare tool: she studied and researched, learning more about her daughter's situation than many of the doctors she visited. She became a discerning reader, keeping a folder of notes and articles in a large binder. Because of her expertise, the doctors look to her for expertise, and she's created phenomenal relationships with the physicians tasked with providing care for her child.

It hasn't been easy, and this mother has certainly gone above the call of duty in terms of healthcare consumerism. It's true that her learning process has consumed her life and required great sacrifice. Advocating for her daughter and her condition has become her mission. As a result, her daughter—who was first diagnosed shortly after birth and considered a candidate for institutional living—has led a full life in her parent's home, including attending school and enjoying many activities typical of the young adult she is.

The mother took control over her daughter's health, learning as much about symptoms and possible solutions as she could, which allowed her to communicate so well that she became an expert herself. In the end, her family was dealt a hand that they didn't think they could play. Instead of folding, though, they responded heroically— thanks, in part, to effective communication.

MEANINGFUL, EVERYDAY SUCCESS

A colleague recently had a DVT (Deep Vein Thrombosis, or a blood clot) that traveled to his lung (making it a pulmonary embolism, or PE). It was a scary, life-threatening event. He also had other complications from previous issues: herniated disc, hip replacement, and arthritis. Each condition required a specialist. While recuperating from the DVT and working with his primary care physician, he wanted to know if there was a connection between the events and conditions. He didn't want the headaches of coordinating and scheduling all those specialists and, most importantly, he wanted a coordinated treatment plan addressing each issue individually and collectively. Therefore, he met with his primary care doctor and went through his specific concerns and goals looking for direction. The PCP advised him to go to an organization that had the expertise and consultative programs in place—in this case, Mayo Clinic, where he received exactly what he was looking for: a team of specialists coordinated by an interfacing lead doctor. The PCP made the referral, and he received the comprehensive consult from a team of specialists at Mayo and was provided an effective coordinated treatment plan.

The bottom line? Your healthcare is not a game. Instead of approaching visits with a chip on your shoulder or with confusion, go in confident and prepared. Build a mutually respectful relationship with them, one in which you communicate openly and concisely. And don't just get to know your doctor; establish relationships with their nurses and their administrative staff, too, because they're the gatekeepers.

If you can build a mutually respectful relationship with your provider, you open the door to negotiate—and negotiations, my friends, can save you some real money.

Here's how to do it.

CHAPTER THIRTEEN

YOU CAN DO IT: BECOMING A HEALTHCARE SHOPPER

So far, we've spent a lot of time preparing, studying, and familiarizing ourselves with who we are health-wise and what options we have. We have a better understanding of the health conditions that may impact our lives, the costs of those services, the profits companies are making on those services, and who is paying for them: YOU. If you're unhappy with your options and escalating costs, what can you do about it? You are paying for all the increases, whether it's through your premium (which seemingly only goes up every year), increased out-of-pocket costs through deductibles, copays, coinsurance, or decreased access. If it were any other consumer good, I'd bet you'd find a way to respond—either boycott or buy alternatives. Yeah, yeah...I know what you're saying, "My healthcare is not a bar of soap or a TV or a car. I'm not willing to challenge individuals entrusted with my care." That's one of the main reasons we are where we are! Up until now, you've been a passive participant in the system. Third parties, insurance carriers, the government, your employer, hospitals, and doctors have been making the decisions for you.

That's about to change. The revolution is going to start with you. I'm not suggesting storming the ramparts and single-handedly taking on one-sixth of the economy. What I'm talking about is taking an active role—one you're entitled to—in the purchasing of your healthcare at the point of service. We'll start small and work on areas that you're comfortable working with and can make a difference in. As your confidence grows through knowledge and practice, you will grow into a healthcare consumer and that will impact your life, and maybe the market. We are all taking baby steps as we go through this process to becoming a smarter consumer of healthcare. The more knowledgeable you are, the more confident you'll be. With that confidence in communication and mutual respect comes one key bonus: you can start to negotiate prices with your healthcare provider.

WHY DO WE CONSUME HEALTHCARE DIFFERENTLY THAN OTHER PRODUCTS WE BUY?

Before we dive into becoming the guru of healthcare negotiation, let's understand why we don't. Common reasons include the following: it's too complicated! Doctors spend years studying, so how can I begin to understand or second-guess them? My insurance company takes care of all that. I don't want to mix money discussions with my health situation; I'm sick and want to get better—that's it! I'm not qualified. I don't know what it costs until after I receive the bill. Doctors never talk about the cost. What if I make a mistake and offend my doctor, my caregiver?

A faculty radiologist at one of the top thirty ranked medical schools in the country added this perspective, "Since the 1950's, medicine had made spectacular advancements: antibiotics, organ transplants, vaccines, birth control in a pill. Medicine became transformative. They were miracle workers. The generations growing up in the fifties, sixties, seventies, and eighties grew to expect miracles from their doctors. You don't question miracles."

But the environment is changing.

Additionally, Quantum's study on a patient's healthcare journey—or, as they call it, "On the Journey Mode"—occurs when someone is sick and has to access the healthcare system.[46] The healthcare journey is unchosen. It is disruptive and potentially life threatening. The resulting stress diminishes cognitive functions, and people begin to have primal emotional responses: fear, freeze, flight, or fight. This is not so far-fetched a concept when you consider that a patient has to make, on average, forty-one decisions through a course of treatment crossing financial, benefit, care, and life issues. How can you advocate on your behalf?

And yet, there continue to be dramatic advances in medicine and genome therapy, intertwining technology into medicine monitoring, identifying and treating conditions earlier, and forming cancer immunotherapies, among a few. What has changed, at its core, is the efficacy of our healthcare system. So many of these procedures incrementally improve our lives, but at what cost? A new report in JAMA published in March of 2018 comparing the US with the highest income countries in the world, points out the US spends far more per capita on healthcare when compared to other countries but has less in healthcare outcomes to show for it. In defense of the US, there are mitigating factors including a more diverse population, freer, quicker access to care, and a litigious environment—but we still spend more on healthcare. We don't ration

---

46 Quantum-health.com. (2018). [online] Available at: https://quantum-health.com/News-Events/Downloads/Quantum-Health-The-Consumers-Journey-112316.pdf [Accessed 21 Sep. 2018].

our healthcare like other nations. Fortunately, the environment is changing in the US. Transparency is driving options and causing the system to reevaluate the efficacy of the treatments being performed. Options are beginning to exist, and it's our job to find them when they do and when they are appropriate, partnering with our providers to find the most cost-effective solutions. President Clinton appointed a commission in 1997 to draft a "consumer bill of rights" for the healthcare industry. Although never fully adopted and subsequently watered down by the American Hospital Association, it directed healthcare professionals to provide consumers with easily understood information and the opportunity to decide among treatment options with an informed consent process. Specifically with regard to treatment and costs it stated:

· Discuss all risks, benefits, and consequences to treatment or non-treatment.
· Give patients the opportunity to refuse treatment and to express preferences about future treatment decisions.
· Disclose to consumers factors—such as methods of compensation, ownership of or interest in healthcare facilities, or matters of conscience—that could influence advice or treatment decisions.

The good news is the budding transparency movement offers the meat to enact those initiatives highlighted in 1997.

So, let's get going.

BASIC CONCEPTS OF HEALTHCARE CONSUMERISM

Let's start with some basic steps on how to become an involved consumer of healthcare.

- Know your objective. Why are you seeing the doctor? Why did you pick that doctor? What do you want to get out of the appointment?
- Be prepared. Do your homework. Who is the right provider to address your issues? Bring your health record. Identify your symptoms in detail. Develop questions. Write them down in a checklist.
- Communicate efficiently and on a factual basis. Remember SBAR.
- Listen with an open mind.
- Ask questions about treatment plan options and cost. Tell them you are paying for the care.
- Don't be afraid to talk about second opinions or seeking alternative cost solutions or cash flow options. Understand how they are paid, by whom, and for how much.
- Research alternatives using the transparency tools and techniques provided. Search for the most cost-effective care.
- Ask again. Reconsult with your caregiver regarding your findings. Solidify a course of action.

- Seek out advocates who can help you organize, listen to, and speak with your caregivers. Look to family, friends, even concierge case managers provided by your health insurance carrier.

ASKING QUESTIONS

As you begin to think about trying to negotiate with providers on cost, remember one key factor: doctors are people, too. They know the pain of paying for healthcare. They are trained to recognize and understand when patients need financial help. Your primary care doctor needs to be involved in your financial wellbeing, and many of them will be—if you ask. Remind them that you're in a High-Deductible Health Plan and are paying out-of-pocket for many of these costs. Here's a list of questions to apply to all categories of caregivers:

- If your diagnosis is complex and treatment is extensive and/or invasive, ask for all available options, their outcomes, and their cost. Ask for referrals of those they successfully treated. Ask for referrals for second opinions.
  - When shopping for alternative care, tap into the transparency tools. Remember costs can vary wildly even in the same city (MRIs from $650 to $1,350 in the same town). Look also regionally and nationally for the best costs and outcomes.

For example, if the average cost for knee replacements in San Francisco is $61,817 versus $27,674 in Detroit, it may be worth your while to travel for the procedure.

- If you're challenged by deductibles, copays, or out-of-pocket costs, ask providers (hospitals/physicians) for payment plans and discounts for paying up front.
  - For example, an individual opted for a High-Deductible Health Plan with an HSA. She had a chronic condition requiring costly monthly medication, which caused short-term cash flow challenges. She went to her physician, and they jointly agreed to a monthly payment plan that stretched her deductible payment over twelve months instead of her having to pay all at once. She was even granted a discount on the amount owed if she paid the last three months at once!
- If your physician is out-of-network, ask them to offset your increased out-of-pocket charges.
  - Doctors and hospitals generally reduce their retail rates by 45 to 50 percent for major health insurance companies. It's worth asking what they'll do for you.
  - Ask if there is a further discount if you pay cash.
- Check the place in which a treatment or procedure is being performed.
  - Outpatient services aren't always less expensive.
  - Diagnostic testing services performed by the

same provider are convenient but often more expensive.

- ◦ Nonprofit hospitals are often less expensive than for-profit while outcomes may be the same.[47]
- ◦ Scrutinize freestanding health facilities. You may think you are at an urgent care facility, but it may be an emergency room extension of a hospital. Charges are significantly different!
- Ask for detailed hospital invoices listing all services upon checkout and look for duplicate charges and services not performed.
  - ◦ Suggestions: if you end up reducing the bill, share your story with your HR department.
  - ◦ If you used an "in-network" hospital and doctor, make sure all the hospital charges are "in-network." Oftentimes, certain medical practices at an "in-network" hospital are actually out-of-network. Thus, they'll cost you significantly more in deductible costs and non-discounted rates. Try to clarify with the hospital how all the charges will be assessed before the treatment. A perfect example is the anesthesiologist. They are often not covered as "in-network" providers and are expensive. Your approach should be that you have complied with the insurance plan and attended an in-network facility that does not make all services available on an in-network basis.

47   Remember, Leapfrog compares these sorts of things. Use them!

How can you be liable for that? Question them: should you have gone to another hospital to have the anesthesiologist perform their service before your surgery at their hospital? Stand your ground with the hospital and the insurance carrier.

- If you have already received care and are now facing unmanageable medical costs, you may want to hire a billing advocate. This type of advocate will normally charge for their services but may be able to save you thousands. They can either charge an hourly rate, generally $100-$200 per hour, or a percentage of the savings from your bill, usually 25-35 percent. You can find patient and medical billing advocates through the National Association of Healthcare Advocacy Consultants or the Alliance of Claims Assistance Professionals.

- Ask for charity care if you're uninsured and at a non-profit hospital.
  - ACA mandates all nonprofit hospitals have a written charity care policy.
  - Individually, you may qualify for discounted or waived charges, depending on the hospital.
  - Regardless, no uninsured individual may be billed for more than the discounted insured rates accepted by the nonprofit hospital.

Again, you don't want to walk into your doctor or hospital and be a belligerent jerk. You are all looking for the best outcome. You have the right to ask questions, and, as you can see, there isn't just one simple, cast-in-stone fee for every service. There is, like any other service industry, a range of options and costs. Remember this and this alone: cash is king. By reducing billing and collection issues, streamlining payments to providers, knowing that discounts are available, and confirming the services billed were performed, you may be able to receive discounts or more favorable treatment. You must ask, research, and audit to achieve.

You may have noticed we did not address pharmacy costs and options. With pharmacy costs fast approaching 50 percent of our healthcare spending, I have dedicated the next chapter to the subject.

CHAPTER FOURTEEN

THE RISING COSTS OF DRUGS

DRUGS: they are everywhere. TV ads are ever-bombarding you with the latest and greatest drug that's going to change your life. They're on every corner. They're in grocery stores. They're available through the mail. Soon, they'll be coming on Amazon! It shouldn't surprise you that seven out of ten Americans are on a prescription drug, that one out of five takes five or more prescriptions at once, or that if you go to a doctor or hospital, you will be prescribed drugs 75 percent of the time.[48] As a result, spending on prescription drugs is increasing and expected to outpace other areas of the healthcare

48   Nearly 7 in 10 Americans Take Prescription Drugs, Mayo Clinic, Olmsted Medical Center Find." Mayo Clinic. Accessed October 25, 2018. https://newsnetwork.mayoclinic.org/discussion/nearly-7-in-10-americans-take-prescription-drugs-mayo-clinic-olmsted-medical-center-find/.

sector in 2018. Projected spending analysis has the prescription drug industry potentially reaching $500 billion in the early twenties.[49]

It's encouraging that medications exist that will address our health issues, but we have become a pill-popping nation. The point here is that the prescription drug industry will probably be your first real experience with the health system, and you need to know something about it because it's not cheap! It can also be the first time you have a choice and can become an involved, informed consumer instead of a passive participant in your healthcare journey. These are the areas you can put into practice being a better consumer and see a real cost impact. Here three examples of the effects of consumerism on the prescription drug industry.

CASE 1: THE RIGHT QUESTIONS CAN LEAD TO THE RIGHT PRICE

Jane had a minor skin cancer on her face and needed a chemical skin peel to remove the precancerous moles. Her dermatologist prescribed Tazorac, a cream that burns off the growths. The two ounces would run $700. She said, "You can't be serious. I have a high-deductible plan

---

49 A Look at Drug Spending in the U.S." The Pew Charitable Trusts. Accessed October 25, 2018. https://www.pewtrusts.org/en/research-and-analysis/fact-sheets/2018/02/a-look-at-drug-spending-in-the-us.

and will be paying for this. Isn't there an alternative?" At that point, the dermatologist put her in touch with a pharmacist company in Pennsylvania that would help out people like her on high-deductible health insurance.

She ended up paying $30 instead of $700—all because she asked questions and had the insight to find an alternative solution.

CASE 2: TRACK RESULTS

An associate was diagnosed with prediabetes and initially prescribed change of diet, weight loss, exercise, and the generic Metformin to treat her condition. After three months, she was making progress on improving her blood sugar average test results, but not to the physician's satisfaction. So, she changed from Metformin to a newer branded, Tradjenta, to improve the results. This was all well and good, but the cost difference was $8/month for Metformin versus $450/month for Tradjenta.

Being an astute consumer, she found a coupon from the manufacture that lowered her cost $150 a month to $300 and began to monitor the effectiveness of the Tradjenta. Then, she searched for alternatives. After three more months and no additional improvement with Tradjenta, she spoke to her doctor about alternatives and discussed that Metformin's dosage could be increased and that could positively affect outcomes. They agreed on altering the treatment again. Happy ending. Her diabetic condition has improved, and she has reduced her cost from $300/month to $30/month.

CASE 3: GET THE BEST PRICE

Two years ago, Jim had a blood clot in his leg which ultimately put him on a blood thinner. The hospital presented him with four options: Warfarin, a generic, and three newer-branded options that did not require the frequent blood tests Warfarin required. Because he did not believe he would be on the thinner for more than a year, he opted for one of the newer-branded, more convenient blood thinners. He asked the hospital pharmacist about the efficacy of the options and chose Eliquis, as it was the cheapest with the same effectiveness. The cost difference was not insignificant—under $10/month at the time versus $380/month.

The pharmacy offered a free month, and he asked if there were any more incentives. They did not respond. Therefore, he contacted the manufacturer and discovered they had a discount program for individuals on High-Deductible Health Plans—of which he was one. The cost went form $380/month to $10/month—the same as Warfarin!

WHAT'S CAUSING THE INCREASE OF UTILIZATION AND COST?

The *Journal of the American Medical Association*'s (JAMA) report on the High Cost of Prescription Drugs in the United States concluded the causes behind the escalating drug costs were a US system that grants pharmaceutical companies twenty-year patent protection (in essence, a monopoly on the drug); the inability of the government health plans (Medicare, Medicaid and Tricare) to negotiate costs or limit the drugs offered under their plans; and physicians' prescription patterns when comparable alternatives are available at different costs.[50] Furthermore, they refute the pharmaceutical companies' assertion that the high costs are due to the extensive research and development required to develop the drugs saying, "There is no evidence of an association between research and development and costs and prices; rather, prescription drugs are priced in the US primarily on the basis of what the market will bear."

There are two impactful takeaways from this report: what the market will bear and what physician prescription patterns present when alternatives are available. Here are three case studies that have something to say about both.

---

50 Kesselheim, A. S., J. Avorn, and A. Sarpatwari. "The High Cost of Prescription Drugs in the United States: Origins and Prospects for Reform." Current Neurology and Neuroscience Reports. Accessed September 26, 2018. https://www.ncbi.nlm.nih.gov/pubmed/27552619.

UNDER ACA, YOUR DOCTOR IS INCENTIVIZED TO MAKE YOU HAPPY

As we statistically illustrated, most interactions you have with the medical community will usually result in you being asked to take a pill. Why? It only makes sense; you go into the doctor expecting to be cured, and you want to walk away with something tangible that tells you you'll get better. Eating right, getting enough sleep, and exercising might fix most people's problems, but that doesn't satisfy them. You also want convenience: one pill per day versus two. What accomplishes this you ask? A prescription.

CASE IN POINT

I worked with a CEO who was facing some health issues due to his lifestyle. This was back when Prilosec, the predecessor of Nexium, was the hot proton pump inhibitor (heartburn medicine) on the market. Doctors were prescribing the expensive drug right and left, and sales skyrocketed. Sure enough, the CEO I was working with got a Prilosec prescription. I told him he didn't have to pop these pills because his was a lifestyle problem; in other words, he could control the problem on his own.

"I gotta have 'em!" he said, animated. "I want to eat my tacos, drink my whiskey, and have my cigars."

His body, however, was clearly rejecting those lifestyle choices, and he was putting a band aid over the problems by taking Prilosec. Eventually, though, he had an epiphany caused by a minor heart incident. He stopped eating tacos, drinking whiskey, and smoking cigars. Lo and behold, he lost weight and never needed another proton pump inhibitor again.

In this case, my client hadn't been looking at the quality of his life. He hadn't been asking if his vices were worth the side effects; he simply accepted them and sought a magic pill to fix the problems they caused, and the system obliged him.

It's important to note that I'm not placing blame here. You don't go into the doctor because you're feeling good; you go in because you feel like crud. If your provider only has eight minutes to make you feel well, and you've been bombarded by advertising claiming miracle cures, you are more than likely going to get a pill. You also might be surprised to learn that under the ACA, part of a doctor's ratings and payment is tied to how a patient feels emotionally after they leave their office, leaving a lot of pressure on the doctor to make you happy. So, if making you happy is writing you a prescription, they are going to do it, and you expect it.

Now, more than ever, those prescriptions are expensive. Specialty drugs, single source branded drugs, and repackaged generic drugs are all escalating in cost (7 percent per year, two times the Consumer Price Index). Remember the EpiPen story? A low-cost generic solution was repurchased and repackaged by Mylan. Then, the drug company increased from $70 to $600 without offering any product enhancements—just price increases! If you aren't aware of how to mitigate those costs, you might be needlessly throwing away thousands of dollars a year. The first step is to understand how they price their drugs and why they're being prescribed.

If you're given a prescription, you should ask the following questions of your doctor *before* committing to taking the drug. Who better to seek advice than Medicare where most of their insureds are taking medication? Medicare recommends the following questions for your doctor:

- What is the name of the medication (both generic and brand name)?
- Why am I taking this medication? What is the name of the condition this medicine will treat?
- Does this medication replace another medication I am currently taking, or should I take it in addition to what I already take?
- Are there any drug interactions to know about? Will the medicine create conflicts with other medicines I take, or will it interact with any of my current health conditions?
- Are there any foods or drinks that the medicine inter-

feres with? Is it okay to eat or drink food before or after I take the medicine? Can I drink alcohol when taking this medicine?

- How will I feel once I start taking this medication?
- How do I take this medication properly? When and how often should I take the medicine? As needed, or on a schedule? Do I take medicine before, with, or between meals? How long will I have to take it?
- What are the benefits of taking this medication?
- What are the risks and side effects I might expect? Should I report them? Are they temporary?
- How long will it take for the medication to work? How will I know if this medication is working?
- How should I store the medicine? Does it need to be refrigerated?
- How much does it cost? Can the pharmacist substitute a cheaper, generic form of the medicine?
- Are there cost-effective alternatives to this medication?
- How many people take the drug? Does it actually help?
- Are there any lab tests to check the medicine's level in my body or for any harmful side effects?
- What should I do if I forget to take it? What if I miss a dose?
- If I want to discontinue taking this medicine, is it safe to just stop?

By asking those questions first, you can determine if your

physician is prescribing something appropriate for you. From there, you can work on reducing your costs.

HOW TO DECREASE DRUG COSTS PRACTICALLY

So, if you and your doctor have agreed on a drug treatment plan, how can you get the best price? SHOP! Here are some suggestions to assist you:

- Turn to big box stores. Wal-Mart, Kroger, Costco, and even Amazon are getting into the drug business. Their goal is to get you in the door (or on the website) by any means necessary. For example, about a decade ago, Wal-Mart accomplished this by selling generic amoxicillin for a mere $4. Consumers came for the dirt-cheap drugs and, while they were there, bought orange juice, milk, and chicken noodle soup. It's a straightforward model, and it still works today; you can find good deals on basic drugs at big box stores.
- Price comparison tools. Check with your insurance plan for such a tool. If you don't have one with your plan or are uninsured, check with the following: GoodRx, One RX, or SingleCare. They all will provide pricing for prescriptions at their negotiated prices. Compare them all. You'll be surprised to find they are different. Also, compare one pharmacy location with one in another area of town. Sometimes there is different pricing, so it pays to look.

- Note: When using one of the discount cards with your health plan, make sure the drug is on your formulary (approved drug list). Research the discount programs for the exact drug. Ask you pharmacist what the cost of the drug is through your health plan. If the discount card is lower, use it instead of your health plan. To receive credit against your deductible, you will need to file that drug as a paper claim. You can access paper claims through your health insurance carriers' web portal. It's worth the extra effort. Check it out.
- Over-the-Counter (OTC) versus Generic; Generic versus brand; Brand versus Brand. Generics are generally cheaper than brands. Unfortunately, you need to be aware of the industry's trend to "patent stack" generics, significantly increasing their price (EpiPen). Therefore, check the over-the-counter alternative. Many times, the prescription for a generic scripted drug is about convenience (for instance, take one pill a day instead of two or four). Remember, you pay for that! Also, check multi-source brand drugs (where there are multiple branded drugs, no generics, treating the same symptom) and determine which has the highest efficacy: best price, similar medical outcome.
- Mail order. If you're on a maintenance drug and your plan offers a mail order program, you may be able to save some money. If your plan has copays for a thirty-day supply, check what the copay is for the mail order at ninety days. It could be less, so it's worth trying.

Also, the mail-order pricing may be more attractive than the retail.

- Volume: buy in bulk. Get your doctor to prescribe a years' worth of maintenance medication versus a thirty- or ninety-day supply, and then shop. Use the highlighted shopping tools for a twelve-month supply. Currently, you can buy a year's supply of atorvastatin, a generic statin heart medicine, for 20 percent less than buying a thirty-day supply each month for a year.
- Volume: buy in higher dosage. Getting a higher dosage and splitting the pill may be less expensive. Ask your doctor, pharmacist, or insurance company if higher dosage and pill splitting would work in your situation.
- Patient Assistance Programs (PAP). RXHOPE is a website that lists over two hundred single source drugs that offer patient assistance programs based on income or for those participating in a high-deductible plan—i.e., 50 percent of the country in 2017. These plans will offer coupons with sometimes dramatic price reductions for a set period of time. I previously highlighted the Eliquis savings, which was through a PAP ($4,440 savings/year). You can also contact the manufacturer of the drug directly and ask for available coupon plans.

Prescriptions drugs are proof that your becoming a better consumer will impact cost. It's the first real cost discussion you'll have with your doctor and one that is nonthreatening to them, as you are not challenging their diagnosis or treatment or questioning their choice of treatment facility. It's a great place to build on your medical consumerism.

HOW DO YOU KNOW IF THESE HIGH-COST DRUGS ARE GOING TO WORK?

Pharmacogenomics, drug-gene testing, is a term used to characterize how your genes affect your body's response to medications. These tests are becoming more prevalent in determining whether or not a drug should be prescribed for an individual. More and more, health plans are covering the cost of the tests on certain drugs and healthcare conditions.

A small amount of saliva or blood can determine:

- Whether a medication may be an effective treatment for you.
- What the best dose of medication is for you.
- Whether you could have serious side effects for a medication.

With the cost of some specialty drugs exceeding $100,000 per complete treatment, and with individuals more and more frequently on multiple medications, it makes sense to understand what drug or drug combination is going to work. Why play trial and error if you don't have to? The tests have been very successful for medications relating to depression and mental health.

Pharmacogenetics is a new and growing area of medicine. It does not cover every situation or drug, but is being increasingly considered and adopted by health plans and doctors. Ask your physician if they have utilized pharmacogenetics and if it should be considered as part of your treatment plan. It may just lead to a better outcome for you.

How else can you reduce your healthcare cost? Don't get sick! We'll explore that in the next chapters.

PART IV

PLANNING AHEAD: START NOW, REAP THE REWARDS LATER

CHAPTER FIFTEEN

AVOIDING HEALTHCARE COSTS ALTOGETHER

Over 50 percent of Americans have at least one chronic condition. Eighty-six percent of healthcare expenditures are a result of chronic diseases. Sixty-seven percent of those expenses are for people under the age of sixty-five. Those two stats might be disheartening, but here's good news: 75 percent of those conditions can be improved or cured by making changes to four aspects of your lifestyle: eating healthy, getting regular exercise, quitting smoking, and reducing stress.[51]

Lifestyle is something you can control. Remember John

---

51 Gerteis, Jessie, David Izrael, Deborah Deitz, Lisa LeRoy, Richard Ricciardi, Therese Miller, and Jayasree Basu. "Multiple Chronic Conditions Chartbook 2010 MEDICAL EXPENDITURE PANEL SURVEY DATA." https://www.ahrq.gov/sites/default/files/wysiwyg/professionals/prevention-chronic-care/decision/mcc/mccchartbook.pdf.

from the beginning of the chapter on Health Risk Assessments? He got off his cholesterol medicine because, through his HRA, he discovered a serious health condition that motivated him to lose 125 pounds. Look, I understand this degree of change is not possible for everyone, as some people have chronic diseases or experience catastrophic events over which they have no control. I get it. I also get something else: catastrophic events represent those made by 2 percent of the population. They're *that* rare. This means when people tell you, "Don't get sick," it's not as ridiculous of a directive as you might think.

When it comes down to it, the best way to lower your healthcare costs is to not get sick in the first place. That, of course, is not always possible—but even when you do get sick, you can look to previous and future lifestyle choices to help you find the best solution.

CASE STUDIES: LIFESTYLE CHANGE FOR THE BETTER

Shirley suffered from debilitating migraines. She tried every doctor and medicine she could find to fix them, but she never found any satisfactory solution. Her medicines would shadow the migraines, but they never completely stopped them. Her life revolved around her condition. To solve her problem, Shirley had to search for her own solutions. Over time, she noticed a correlation between her migraines and her consumption of dairy products.

She didn't know if there was anything to it, but she tried an experiment on her own and stopped consuming dairy. It worked! It turned out she had a food allergy she didn't know about. Just like that—no more doctors. No more medicine. No more migraines.

Steve—only thirty-one years old—had herniated his L3, L4, and L5 discs in his back. At first, doctors told him to take a couple aspirin for the pain. Eventually, their recommendations progressed to him getting an MRI and saying he needed immediate surgery to fuse his vertebrae. Steve almost said yes (because, after all, these were doctors, right?). Thankfully, he took a step back and looked at the whole picture, considering the long-term implications of his next choice. He talked to athletes who'd had the same surgery at the same age. Through his research, he discovered that fusing the vertebrae, especially that low on his back, puts stress on the rest of his vertebrae. The people he spoke to had to go back for surgery after surgery after surgery over time as the rest of their back eventually broke down.

He found that when people were honest about the complications of back surgery, they recommended he only consent to the procedure if the pain got so bad he couldn't stand it. In short, his peers who had been there before told him surgery should be a last resort. These tough conversations made Steve consider whether he could change his health outcomes by changing his life-style, and he began looking into alternatives to surgery. Ultimately, he chose a type of physical therapy focused on strengthening his core as an alternative to full-fledged back surgery. No, physical therapy didn't make his back perfect, but it didn't impede his daily duties or his ability to exercise the same way the surgery would have. Like-wise, he avoided about $70,000 in healthcare costs. More importantly, he got a better overall health outcome based on his sense of alternatives as an individual.

PREEMPTIVE STRIKES AGAINST ILLNESS

The healthcare industry is focused more on reacting to problems rather than being preventive. It is set up to help you with acute, specific issues. I'm asking you to take a step back and look at your health holistically. Holistic medicine means thinking about you, the whole person; your physical and mental health, as well as the environment in which you live. Become proactive. It's your responsibility to take care of your greatest asset: YOU. Working daily on you and your health just makes good sense. You could argue that if you are genetically pre-disposed to a health condition—like heart disease, the number one killer of Americans, you are destined for heart issues.[52] Instead, think of it this way: "What you

---

52   Healthline. (2018). *12 Leading Causes of Death in the United States.* [online] Available at: https://www.healthline.com/health/leading-causes-of-death [Accessed 26 Sep. 2018].

do and how you live is going to have a larger impact on whether you are in ideal cardiovascular health than your genes or how you were raised," said Norrina Allen, the lead study author and a postdoctoral fellow in preventive medicine at the Feinberg School. The Northwestern University study looked at three generations of families from all walks of life.[53] So, it just makes sense to manage your lifestyle. We can always point the blame at someone else or look toward others for our solutions instead of looking to ourselves. You, your choices, and your actions can truly make a difference.

Avoiding healthcare costs might take you down different paths. Like Steve and his back pain, you might find ways to work within the healthcare industry to find a less drastic solution to your ailment. Like Sheila and her migraines, you might find the answer in a small change to your daily routine.

There's a wellness craze in this country at the moment, but people still get sick. Why? Because the hard work it takes to stay healthy is not sexy, simple, or quick. Even if people are motivated to change—when they have all the resources and knowledge to do so—they still want quick solutions. "I've got too much going on in my life," they'll say. "Just give me the pill." You could tell people to eat

53   "News." Northwestern University. Accessed September 26, 2018. https://www.northwestern. edu/newscenter/stories/2010/11/heart-disease.html.

right and get exercise until you're blue in the face, but it doesn't mean they'll actually do it.

There have to be material consequences to motivate people to take preemptive strikes against illness through lifestyle changes. If not, you at least need personal reasons to be motivated. For example, if you're a smoker and have three kids, you might want to see them all go through college and get married. You can't be there at those major life events if you're dead. Maybe you see a close friend who's a smoker die, and you say to yourself, "I have to quit." There has to be a catalyst that prompts you to change; you can't just read the literature.

Overall, the world is moving to coddle people more. Health plans are more willing to reward you for taking actions you should be taking anyway; they're realizing they have to make it worth something to you. They'll give you discounts if you eat right, exercise, and keep your weight down. Employers don't want employees complaining about pain and getting sick all the time, so the relationship between health and work has changed, too.

This lecture doesn't apply to everyone; I know there are different degrees of sickness. If you're healthy, you can continue to do what you're doing. If you're sick but not seriously sick, you can look at your life holistically and take these measures to improve your situation. If you're seriously sick, you can still try these solutions, but you won't find any miracle cures. For example, if you have stage four cancer, eating right and exercising won't in and of itself cure you—but it can help.

What's it going to take to get you off the proverbial couch and be proactive with your health? The results from your Health Risk Assessment you took in chapter 3? An annual physical? A health scare? A friend or family member's illness? A marriage? The birth of a child? A divorce? The death of a family member? Just a desire to feel better? Whatever it is, this is how you can change your health.

A FOOD PARADIGM SHIFT

In our society, food equals pleasure, entertainment, breaks from our daily monotonous routine, communal experiences, or—said differently—nonnutritional factors. We need to reintroduce the proper purpose of food: to efficiently fuel our bodies. I know there are tons of diet plans bombarding your every waking moment; there are TV personalities peddling testimonials, books, tapes, spas, and wellness programs. The diet business is a billion-dollar industry, but—let's face it—habits and practices are near impossible to break!

What if those habits are literally making you sick and costing you potentially enormous amounts of money and your health? If you went to your doctor and he gave you a nutritional pill to treat your illness, wouldn't you take it? With the costs you're going to face in the healthcare system and insurance, you should try to do everything you can.

Everyone has their own unique DNA. No one diet will be right for everyone but finding the right one can alleviate or eliminate illness. Diesel fuel in a gas engine will trash that engine, and we are no different. Remember Shirley and her migraines?

Are you wondering how to start? Use your Health Risk Assessment and health records to see who you are. Consult with your primary care doctor, dietician, or qualified health coach about a specific diet that is right for you. When you feel off, track what you've been eating. See if a pattern and correlation present itself. Mayo Clinic and the FDA have put out guidelines that are worth considering, testing, and trying. The word "diet" has such a negative and short-term connotation. Instead, think of it as lifestyle. What's our perception of how Italians, Greeks, and the provincial French eat? I don't know about you, but those lifestyles are pretty attractive to me. Guess what? They are the original Mediterranean diet touted by so many diet resources. So, *Vita Longa*!

HOW ABOUT THIS FOR MOTIVATION

Dr. Stephen Messier's study appearing in the July 2005 *Journal of Arthritis & Rheumatism* concluded that for every one pound of weight loss that occurred, there was a resulting four-pound reduction in knee joint load or knee pressure.[54] Furthermore, it was suggested that individuals who lost ten pounds would be subject to a total of 48,000 less pounds of pressure for every mile walked. Multiply this change in workload over an average lifespan, and you get a compelling case for weight loss as an approach to alleviate knee pain in individuals who are overweight or obese.

You are what you eat, but did you ever consider that what you eat is what it eats? I am admittedly a foodie. I love to cook and try new things. I have become obsessed with concocting full mouth experiences without feeling stuffed. I also suffer from advanced arthritis and am constantly looking for foods that will minimize inflammation. To that end, my studies have come across two books of interest that I pass along: *The Omnivore's Dilemma* by Michael Pollan and *The Dorito Effect* by Mark Schatzker. Both address the diminished nutritional value of the food

---

54 Messier, S. P., D. J. Gutekunst, C. Davis, and P. DeVita. "Weight Loss Reduces Knee-joint Loads in Overweight and Obese Older Adults with Knee Osteoarthritis." Current Neurology and Neuroscience Reports. July 2005. Accessed September 26, 2018. https://www.ncbi.nlm.nih.gov/pubmed/15986358.

we eat today. You can't just follow the proper diet; you need to know how that diet was produced.

The Omnivore's Dilemma uses four separate eating experiences, starting with the soils in which the produce (fruits, vegetables, and grains) grew or the feed the proteins (chicken, beef, pork, turkey) ate and ends up with a cooked finished meal. It compares the calories it took to produce the meal versus the calories and nutritional value of consuming each meal. The meals are as follows: a meal from McDonalds; a meal prepared with ingredients from Whole Foods grocery store; an organic chicken dinner from a self-sustaining farm in Virginia that does not use pesticides, antibiotics, or synthesized fertilizers; and a hunter-gatherer feast consisting almost entirely of ingredients shot or foraged by one individual.

As you might imagine, the results are predictable. Organic, more natural, raised or grown ingredients used in meals were more flavorful and more satiating. The truly fascinating part, though, is the detailed explanation of where food comes from and the history and dominance of corn in almost every aspect of agribusiness. It is important to understand that most of the livestock we get our protein from is fed an unnatural diet consisting mostly of corn and other grains. Therefore, when we eat chicken, we really are consuming more and more starch than protein. How do you think chicken breasts have gotten so big? I think we all know just eating starches leads to obesity, which leads to heart, cancer, and joint problems. If you interested in getting the book, look for the updated tenth anniversary edition.

The Dorito Effect dives down in to the science of flavor—natural flavor and the creation of flavor through science. The author highlights historically how the food industry has focused on producing more of something and how it looks versus how it tastes. Think about it: Why do those gorgeous, huge tomatoes at the grocery store taste like paste? Why does deli turkey taste nothing like a free-range roasted turkey?

Flavor, the author asserts and supports, is nutrition. Our bodies are wired to seek out the flavor—aka nutritional values—and consume them until satisfied. The problem with the synthetically raised produce is that it doesn't have those flavor markers, so our bodies still crave the nutrients. Hence, we eat more and gain weight without ever really satisfying the nutrient needs.

What's inherent to both of their assertions is eating natural wholesome foods. Processed foods are not preferable. Check labels. If you can't pronounce the ingredients, they probably aren't the best for you. The overabundance of preservatives, fat, sugar, and salt in all processed foods blow away our daily requirements. Here's the dilemma:

fat, sugar, and salt are the base that give most food dishes their pop. Therefore, they are in almost everything. Understand what you're eating. Managing the levels of those ingredients will dramatically affect not only your weight, but also how you feel.

FARM-TO-TABLE MOVEMENT

Food matters to your health because, to a certain extent, you are what you eat. A New York chef named Dan Barber is taking that axiom to heart. He's working with Cornell University, among others, to create high-nutrient, high-flavored foods. Whereas most grocery stores and distributors focus on trying to get the biggest chickens and biggest fruits and vegetables farmers can produce, Dan wants the most flavor possible. He experimented by feeding chickens hot peppers, for example. Lo and behold, the yolk in their egg was spicy.

He even wrote a book about it called The Third Plate: Field Notes on the Future of Food. Dan is at the forefront of a farm-to-table movement that is focused on locally grown, in-season food. He focuses on food that's smaller and more flavorful, which nature has told us is a sign that it's more nutritious.

What's my point? There are beacons of light out there providing healthier alternatives. You can find them in farmers markets, restaurants, certain grocery stores. On the path to taking preemptive strikes against illness, looking at the food you eat is a good place to start. Know what you are eating!

EXERCISE: YOU HAVE TO KEEP MOVING

The human race was not designed to be stationary. We were hunters and gatherers. In other words, we moved all the time. Dan Buettner, founder of "Blue Zones," studied five locations across the world: Okinawa, Japan; Sardinia, Italy; Ikaria (a small island off of Turkey); and a seventh-day adventist community in Northern California and Costa Rica, where living past one hundred years was not uncommon. Buettner contends that scientists have determined the average physical capabilities of the human body max out at ninety years. Then, he observed the average US life span is seventy-eight years. How are they gaining twelve additional quality years of life? Why were these communities experiencing people living beyond one hundred?

He found strong correlations of lifestyle that included a sense of personal connection with the community, a purpose in life, a primarily vegetarian diet with plenty of beans, and lots of low intensity, constant physical activity.[55]

---

55   For more, visit For more www.bluezones.com.

Note that movement was a key factor, not just for becoming an Olympic athlete, marathon runner, or someone who spends every waking hour in the gym. This proves changing your life to move more can have substantial impact. Walking up the steps instead of the escalator or elevator, walking or riding a bike to the store versus driving, walking the dog, or standing instead of sitting at your desk, are all seemingly minor lifestyle changes you can do and have a substantial impact on your health and life. Find a reason to move!

CASE IN POINT

Dan was seventy-five and diagnosed with atrial fibrillation, a heart condition. He was put on the requisite medications and was placed on a six-month visitation schedule. His conditioned stabilized, and life went on under the course of treatment. Sometime later, he got a dog, and he got into a routine of walking that dog a mile or two at least and sometimes twice per day. Soon afterward, at one of his six-month checkups, his cardiologist informed him that his heart condition had improved enough that he wouldn't need to come in every six months but every two years. All that from a dog!

The CDC and the medical community support Dan's experiences. They state that regular physical activity is one of the most important things you can do for your health. Here are areas research has found physical activity improves your health, according to the aforementioned resource from the CDC:

- Control your weight
- Reduce your risk of cardiovascular disease
- Reduce your risk of Type 2 diabetes and metabolic syndrome
- Reduce your risk of some cancers
- Strengthen your bones and muscles
- Improve your mental health and mood
- Improve your ability to do daily activities and prevent falls
- Increase your chances of living longer

Just like diet programs, there is no lack of exercise programs that promise to transform you and your life. I'm not telling you anything new. It works because it's who we are. Movement can and should be incorporated into your daily life. A mere two-hour to two-and-a-half-hours per week or twenty minutes per day will make a difference for a sedentary person's weight, blood pressure, cholesterol, and blood sugar. It can also slow the loss of bone density, relieve painful joints, reduce injuries and broken bones, decrease the chance of colon and breast cancer, enhance your immune system, reduce inflammation, and improve your mental health.

Who of you do not associate with one of those conditions on the list? Exercise/movement is a great medicine in helping to manage them—and it's free! As you progress your physical activity, work on maintaining muscle tone and a strong core. Core muscles, muscles in your pelvis, back, hips, and abdomen, provide your body with balance and stability, supporting your back and skull. Anyone who's experienced back pain knows how debilitating it can be.

Reach out to your doctor and ask for resources in developing an appropriate physical activity program. You don't have to belong to a gym. Comprehensive programs can be designed for your personal situation and environment utilizing ordinary everyday items. Check out yoga, Tai Chi, or stretching programs. If motivation is an issue, find a group to work out with. Find a way to get off the couch. You'll thank yourself in the end!

MENTAL HEALTH AND SPIRITUALITY

One thing is apparent to anyone who has either been seriously or chronically ill or has been around those who are: being ill affects mental health. Anxiety, depression, and mood swings all accompany physical illness. Similarly, poor mental health leads to poor physical health. The Mental Health Foundation in England reports on various ways mental health affects physical health.[56] They have found a 67 percent increased risk of death from heart disease and a 50 percent risk of death from cancer.

Familydoctor.org expands further: when stressful events happen in life, like job loss, the death of a loved one, divorce, money problems, or moving, physical manifestations show up in higher blood pressure and stomach ulcers. Over extended periods of time, both contribute heavily to serious physical issues.

Dan Buettner's findings found purpose of life and a personal sense and involvement in community were instrumental in promoting a centurion lifestyle in the communities he studied. The Mayo Clinic has found correlations with spirituality and Dan's community observations. They define spirituality as a belief system and approach to life that gives your life context, a value system, and meaningful connection with others. Being in good emotional health allows us to clearly be aware of our own thoughts, feelings, and behaviors, granting us the ability to cope with stress.

---

56 "Physical Health and Mental Health." Mental Health Foundation. August 27, 2018. Accessed September 21, 2018. https://www.mentalhealth.org.uk/a-to-z/p/physical-health-and-mental-health.

MANAGING STRESS

Stress exacerbates illness. Ninety percent of primary care visits, in fact, have some relationship to stress.[57] Why? Chronic stress can suppress your immune system, diminish your judgment, and squash your coping abilities. What happens when you combine all of those factors? You wind up feeling sick and making bad decisions right when you need your strength and good judgment the most.

Many people cope with stress in negative ways. Forty-three percent of people, according to the Mayo Clinic, turn to overeating. Thirty percent of people skip meals, and 39 percent of people drink alcohol to cope with stress. Turning these choices around is all about habits; you can create a vicious cycle that exacerbates stress. Often times, people have a tendency to gravitate to others who share the same struggles, which often only fosters negative commiseration. The old adage "misery loves company" holds true here. Or, you can cope with stress by forming healthy habits. For example, exercise, listening to music, reading, and spending time with friends are all healthy coping mechanisms. You can also pray, meditate, do yoga, or focus on other transcendental practices. You can even try alternative therapies, such as acupuncture, massage, and the chiropractic therapies.

---

57   "Plato and Aristotle on Health and Disease." Psychology Today. Accessed June 25, 2018. https://www.psychologytoday.com/us/blog/hide-and-seek/201203/plato-and-aristotle-health-and-disease?amp.

NO YOGI

I'm so inflexible that when I tried yoga, it just about killed me. I was sandwiched between two young kids who downward-dogged with ease. Meanwhile, I was sweating so much it looked like Niagara Falls dripping down onto my mat. I felt like the instructor was telling us to put our left foot behind our right ear, and I just couldn't keep quiet anymore. I blurted out, "Oh, you have got to be kidding me," and ruined all serenity and peace in the room.

Yoga is not for everyone—but hey, at least I tried!

For additional assistance, explore approaches by professionals like Dr. Frank Wood or Ryan Luke Seaward. Dr. Frank Wood has a PhD in clinical psychology and created a program called "Thriving with Stress." His premise is that stress is not what happens *to* us; rather, it is in our responses. It is this "stress response" that is both helpful in the short term and yet damaging to us if it persists. Those who learn to leverage the energy that comes with stressful circumstances tend to find a way to be productive, while those who endeavor to avoid, contain, or control those challenges tend to become "stressed out."

Ryan Luke Seaward, an international expert in the field of stress, created a company called Inspiration Unlimited Paramount Wellness Institute and teaches people how to manage their stress in a healthy way. My point is there are many people out there with stress management tools to help you, so it's time to listen.

RECHARGING YOUR BATTERY

We'd all like to be like Energizer Bunny, going and going—but we don't run on batteries. Coffee and energy drinks may appear to keep us "ever ready," but they don't allow us to recharge. We need sleep to recharge. The medical community is finding deeper correlations between adequate sleep and health conditions. Harvard University's Division of Sleep Medicine at Harvard Medical School found that numerous studies have shown that "insufficient sleep increases a person's risk for developing serious medical conditions including obesity, diabetes, and cardiovascular disease."

Here are some of their findings:[58]

- Obesity: fewer than six hours per night is more likely to have excess body weight and reduced metabolism. People with eight hours had less body fat.
- Diabetes: fewer than five hours/night increased risk of type 2 diabetes. Good news: improved sleep can positively reduce the effects of type 2 diabetes.

---

58 "Sleep and Disease Risk." Benefits of Sleep | Healthy Sleep. Accessed September 26, 2018.
    http://healthysleep.med.harvard.edu/healthy/matters/consequences/sleep-and-disease-risk.

- Cardiovascular disease and hypertension: even modestly reduced sleep, five to seven hours/night, was associated with greater increase of artery calcification and death from heart disease.
- Immune function: sleep deprivation increases the levels of many inflammatory conditions and increases infections.
- Death: three independent studies concluded sleeping less than five hours/night increases mortality 15 percent.

If you're not sleeping well, address the issue. It's worth your time!

Ultimately, your mind, body, and spirit all need to be in healthy alignment in order to stay healthy. If that means you need to go to an acupuncturist three days a week, start working out every day, growing your own food, and do stress-relieving yoga every week, then more power to you. More than likely, though, it'll mean you take a look at your current stress levels and see how you can work with them without the unrealistic expectation of dissolving them completely. It'll mean watching what you eat and getting consistent exercise. And it will mean breaking bread with friends and family to rejuvenate your spirit. With all of those things in alignment, through baby steps, you'll start to create a virtuous cycle in your life, rather than a vicious one.

CHAPTER SIXTEEN

RETIREMENT PLANNING

You may be thinking: What are you talking about? That's Medicare!

Nope. You need to realize that Medicare does not eliminate your medical expenses once you hit sixty-five. There are premium payments, deductibles, and coinsurance just like your current health coverage and, like your current coverage, those features cost more every year. The sooner you can get your mind, body, and spirit aligned, the better off you'll be in retirement. I can't neglect the elephant in the room: part of that alignment is getting your financial situation taken care of. Many of us unwittingly walk into our retirement years thinking, "Oh my god—I can't afford this!" The solution is to face your financial situation dead on, make an assessment, and take the responsibility to change what you need to change.

Retiree medical costs need to be included in your long-term financial planning.

Here's why: you've contributed to Medicare through a payroll tax all the years you've worked. Those contributions and the premiums you pay once on Medicare should cover expenses. The problem is people are living longer than anticipated, and medical advancements, a large contributor to longevity gains, are costlier. Couple that with a Medicare population that will increase 20 percent as a percentage of the total population between 2016 and 2030, a national debt that is approaching our GDP, and a Social Security System facing similar issues, and it's reasonable to assume Medicare participant costs are going to go up.[59]

Wondering how much you need to save? A 2016 report by EBRI[60] proports that to cover program deductibles, premiums for Medicare Parts B, D, a Medigap Plan F, and out-of-pocket costs for prescription drugs, a man would need to save $127,000 and a woman $143,000 to cover 90 percent of those costs. It would be unwise to rely on the cost of living adjustments extended to social security

59   15, 2013 Jul. "Projected Change in Medicare Enrollment, 2000-2050." The Henry J. Kaiser Family Foundation. July 17, 2013. Accessed June 25, 2018. https://www.kff.org/medicare/slide/projected-change-in-medicare-enrollment-2000-2050/.

60   "EBRI.org Notes: Savings Medicare Beneficiaries Need for Health Expenses: Some Couples Could Need as Much as $350,000." *EBRI Notes* 38, no. 1 (January 31, 2017). https://www.ebri.org/pdf/notespdf/EBRI_Notes_Hlth-Svgs.v38no1_31Jan17.pdf.

payments. In many cases, the Medicare increases take disproportional amounts of the increase.[61] The situation can be disheartening, to say the least. Still, though, it's best to look at the facts.

GET A HEAD START

If you can factor retirement healthcare costs into your retirement planning sooner rather than later, you'll be better off. To put that advice into perspective, saving an additional $100 per month per person over thirty years using a 7.9 percent historical US stock market return would cover the anticipated retiree's medical out-of-pocket costs.[62] Talk to a financial advisor, accountant, or insurance agent, and ask them if they factor in retiree healthcare costs in their projections. If not, why not? Have them present their firm's calculations on the costs. The AARP is a good place to seek advice. They have calculators projecting retiree healthcare costs. Here are the best ways to do it: take advantage of any and all tax-deferred savings plans available.

---

61   Miller, Mark. "Column: Big Social Security COLA Will Be Offset by Medicare Premiums." Reuters. June 22, 2017. Accessed June 25, 2018. https://www.reuters.com/article/us-column-miller-socialsecurity-idUSKBN19D1J0.

62   Standard disclosure regarding results may vary check with you advisor. Your actual results may be different results. Historical data is not a predictor to future results.

- Max out your 401(k), 403(b), or 457 plans ($18,500 under fifty and $24,500 over fifty for 2018).[63]
- Max out your Health Savings Account (HSA). Max individual contribution $3,450 and $6,900 for family coverage.
- Fund IRAs. You can contribute annually up to $5,500 or $6,500 if over fifty.

All contributions are pre-tax, and earnings in the funds are tax deferred. Whatever tax advantage situation applies to you, it's the best way to save.

BREAK OUT THE BUNNY EARS

Pam is quite austere, using bunny ears to get television and using Netflix for anything else. Now, that may seem extreme, but she's easily saving the $100/month she needs to save for retiree healthcare costs. Unfortunately, healthcare costs' impact on our lives requires us missing a few television stations, expensive coffee, celebrity-endorsed athletic shoes, or larger TVs, but that isn't going to kill you. Not having enough retirement savings might.

---

63 "IRS Announces 2018 Pension Plan Limitations; 401(k) Contribution Limit Increases to $18,500 for 2018." Internal Revenue Service. Accessed June 25, 2018. https://www.irs.gov/newsroom/irs-announces-2018-pension-plan-limitations-401k-contribution-limit-increases-to-18500-for-2018.

CONCLUSION

Are you mad as hell about the state and costs of healthcare but still sitting on your butt, not doing anything to take charge of your physical health or your role in your own care? That stops now. I've covered lots of information in this book, but if you take nothing else away, take this: we're talking about *your* health and *your* dollars, so act like it. Be possessive! Be aggressive! Start developing an understanding of healthcare and insurance until you see improved outcomes in your own life.

Look, you can't fully avoid all medical events in life. You're going to get sick in some capacity at some point, and we both know it. When those situations arise, your goal should be to do everything you can to minimize their negative impact on you physically and financially. If this book helps you do just a little bit of that—and, hopefully, provides you with incentive to educate and motivate yourself around your health situation—I will have accomplished my task.

Remember one thing: healthcare is a consumer good, and you're a consumer. *Understand* that. *Repeat* that. *Teach* it to everyone you know. Practice, practice, practice being a consumer. When it comes to your healthcare, know why you want it, when you want it, and how you want it. Ask questions: Who are the best service providers? What are the best products out there? Who's giving the best deals? Demand transparency and a certain level of service from every medical professional you come into contact with. You need to hold them accountable, the same way you would anybody else. Do you allow your car mechanic to do anything and everything to your car that he suggests? Should you with anyone? Let alone when it comes to your health? The apathy ends today.

The healthcare industry's transparency is in its embryonic stage, but the information is out there if you know where to find it. The shell of the egg has cracked, and data is starting to flow out. Gather the information yolk and share it with others. Here's the thing: exposure of outcomes and cost is bringing about change. Amazon, Berkshire Hathaway, and Chase Bank have said enough is enough. The EpiPen story proves cost exposure and your voices can bring about change. Think about the impact the #MeToo movement is having with subject matter heretofore untouchable. Transparency and technology are changing the healthcare profession. Let's use it to our advantage as an empowered consumer looking out for our best interests. As you improve your life and health at better costs, you'll be taking part in a change in the industry. Share your stories and watch a collection of small changes spark a revolution.

You've probably heard the saying, "The definition of insanity is doing the same thing over and over again and expecting a different outcome." Turn that premise on its head when it comes to your healthcare and stop accepting your own lack of understanding. Ask for what you want from this industry. Hold service providers accountable by asking them questions. If they're good at what they do, it can start a dialogue between you two, and all the sudden, there's a back and forth between doctor and patient. The result? You get the best care possible, and you don't go broke doing it. And, by sharing your journey, you can become an advocate for others.

At the end of the day, the only guarantee in this life is that everything will change. If you're tired of being mad as hell at the healthcare and insurance system, the time to stand up is now. The worst thing that can happen is that you have a better understanding of yourself, the marketplace, and its related costs.

I know as well as anyone that the industry changes daily. That's why I've created **Uncoveredhc.com**—to capture everything you need to know to guide you along your journey. It's time to stop being mad as hell, start improving your healthcare outcomes, and—of course—save money. Visit us, add your stories, tell us what you need, and let's move the needle forward together.

What do you have to lose?

UNCOVEREDHC.COM REFERENCE GUIDE

PHYSICIANS

CUSTOMER SERVICE REVIEWS

- WebMD.com
- Yelp
- Healthgrades.com
- RateMDs.com
- Vitals.com
- Caredash.com

COST AND OUTCOMES

- Aminohealth.com
- Guroo.com
- Healthcarebluebook.com
- Castlight.com

PHYSICIAN CONCIERGE SERVICES

- MDVP.com
- Pinnacle.com

PRESCRIPTION DRUGS

- GoodRx.com
- OneRx.com
- SingleCare.com
- RxHope.com

INSURANCE

GOVERNMENT

- Medicare.gov
- Medicaid.gov
- American Council on Aging's Medicaid resources medicaidplanningassistance.org
- Children's Health Insurance Program (CHIP)
- 1-800-318-2596
- Healthcare.gov

PRIVATE MEDICAL

- Anthem
- Aetna
- Blue Cross Blue Shield organizations
- Cigna
- Kaiser Permanente

PRIVATE SUPPLEMENTAL MEDICAL

- Aflac

- Colonial Life Insurance Company
- Principal Financial Group
- American Fidelity
- Assurant Life insurance Co

COMBINED INSURANCE

- AIG
- Aetna
- Cigna
- Humana
- Blue Cross Blue Shield
- United Healthcare

HOSPITALS

- Leapfrog.com
- Medicare.gov

MEDICAL TOURISM

- PatientsBeyondBorders.com

HEALTH EDUCATION
GENERAL

- Mayoclinic.com
- Clevelandclinic.com
- American Council on Aging

- Centers for Disease and Control and Prevention Presentation, CDC.gov
- Agency for Healthcare Research and Quality AHQR Division of the Dept. of HHS, ahrq.gov

STRESS

- Unlimited Paramount Wellness Institute, Brian Luke Seaward Ph.D.
- Thriving with Stress, Frank Wood

HOLISTIC

- Bluezones.com
- Harvard University's Division of Sleep Medicine at Harvard Medical School

RELIGIOUS

- SamaritanMinistries.com
- Christianhealthcareministires.com
- Medishare.com
- Libertyhealthshare.com
- Unitedrefuahhs.org

ADMINISTRATIVE
GENERAL

- Healthcare.gov
- Healthsherpa.com
- Irs.gov Publication 502, Qualified Medical and Dental Expenses
- Kaiser Family Foundation KFF.org
- AARP.com

BILLING ADVOCATES

- The Alliance of Claims Assistance Professionals
- Association of Healthcare Advocacy Consultants
- Broken Healthcare

FINANCIAL ASSISTANCE

- Patient Access Network Foundation
- Patient Services
- Health Well Foundation
- Cancer Care
- American Cancer Society
- Leukemia and Lymphoma Society (financial aid program)
- Needy Meds
- Patient Advocate Foundation
- American Kidney Fund

ACKNOWLEDGMENTS

To my wife, for her encouragement, advice, guidance, and support. You are my rock.

To Carol, Monica, Mike, Cris, Marge, Brent, Frank, Nancy, Beth, Ken, and Jeff, who provided expertise, insight, and personal experiences that make the book what it is.

And, to Jessica Burdg, who guided me through this journey and helped shape its outcome.

CPSIA information can be obtained
at www.ICGtesting.com
Printed in the USA
LVHW031551061119
636549LV00002B/322